Baby Boomer's Guide to Women's Health

LIVING GREAT
THE NEXT 50 YEARS

KARLA DOUGHERTY
& RICHARD C. SENELICK, MD

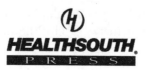

HEALTHSOUTH
PRESS

This book is not intended to replace personal medical care and/or professional supervision; there is no substitute for the experience and information that your doctor or healthcare professional can provide. Rather, it is our hope that this book will provide additional information to help women of all ages live healthier and happier lives.

If you read something in this book that seems to conflict with any of your doctors or healthcare professionals' instructions, contact them. There may be sound reasons for recommending behavior that may differ from the information presented in this book.

If you have any questions about any treatment or suggestions in this book, please consult your doctor or healthcare professional.

Also, the names and cases used in this book do not represent actual people, but are composite cases drawn from several sources.

Library of Congress Catalog Card Number 2001132823
ISBN: 1-891525-11-5
First HealthSouth Printing
10 9 8 7 6 5 4 3 2
HealthSouth Press and colophon are registered trademarks of HealthSouth
Printed in Canada

THE FACTS ABOUT HEALTHSOUTH

HealthSouth Corporation is the nation's largest physical rehabilitation healthcare provider with more than 100,000 patients being treated in its facilities every day.

The HealthSouth network includes rehabilitation hospitals and acute-care medical centers, as well as outpatient rehabilitation, ambulatory surgery, and diagnostic imaging centers. Some of its diverse services include the treatment of spinal cord injury, sports injuries, brain injury, stroke, pain management, oncology rehabilitation, geriatric rehabilitation, and such diagnostic services as mammography, magnetic resonance imaging (MRI), nuclear medicine, and ultrasound.

HealthSouth Press has been created to help patients and their families understand the ramifications of their injury or illness. All of its books are written to help families learn how to cope with life's unexpected changes. And, above all, each book is designed to show, in compassionate and intelligent terms, that you, the reader, are not alone.

ℐCKNOWLEDGMENTS

We would like to thank Richard Scrushy, Pat Foster, Brad Hale and Gerald Nix of HealthSouth for their continued support and help in making HealthSouth Press a success. We would also like to thank Gray Richardson, Tim Robinson, and the entire art staff of HealthSouth Press for their talent, expertise, and hard work. We also want to thank Patricia Brown of HealthSouth RIOSA for keeping things running smoothly.

We would also like to thank the following specialists who took time away from their work to ensure that the information in these pages is not only accurate, but as cutting edge as possible: Dr. Claudia Hura, Dr. Haskel Hoine, Dr. John King, Dr. Jerome Fischer, Dr. George Lowry, Dr. Charles Roeth, Dr. Tim Hlavinka, Dr. Carolyn Cavazos, Dr. Wesley Krueger, Dr. Mark Weinstein, and Dr. Jorge Munoz.

DEDICATION

To women everywhere. May the information in this book point you in healthier, happier, and more informed directions as you age.

☾ABLE OF CONTENTS

Calling All Baby Booming and Still Blooming Women

Getting old? Not Susan! She might have turned 53 in September, but, inside, where it counts, she was only 24. Her memory was sharp, her face was still fairly smooth, and, thanks to a daily regime of healthy food, exercise, and a good night's sleep, her body was still slim.

But about three weeks ago, something happened. She suddenly noticed her stomach; it bulged. She didn't get her period. The lines on her face looked a bit more pronounced. She sometimes needed people to repeat what they'd just said. She squinted when she tried to read the newspaper.

Susan started to panic. "This isn't happening to me!" She started exercising with a vengeance, ignoring her family and her real estate job. She shook her head at desserts and wine, even on her birthday. She started interviewing plastic surgeons and she gobbled tons of nutritional supplements whose names she couldn't even pronounce.

But as the months passed, Susan continued to squint when she had to read small print. She still couldn't hear properly. Her menstrual cycle was still irregular. And she sometimes had a "senior moment"—forgetting an appointment she'd made earlier that day.

Susan refused to give in. She became obsessed with youth. She quit her job and spent four hours a day at the gym. She ignored her family's complaints and made dinners that consisted only of dry fish, raw vegetables, and plain yogurt shakes. She spent a small fortune on dietary supplements—from digestive enzymes to blue algae tablets. She ran to the dermatologist for implants and chemical peels the way other people go to the movies. She scheduled a tummy tuck and laser eye surgery, and she took natural *and* prescription hormones to ward off her menopause symptoms.

But Susan still had trouble remembering certain things. She still grew tired in the afternoon. She still had more frequent headaches, more aches and pains.

Why? What was Susan doing wrong? Nothing.

Aging, like taxes and unwanted facial hair, is a fact of life. We are getting older. In fact, today there are 31 million people over the age of 65 *nationwide*. But the survival rate of people between the ages of 65 and 74 is eight times higher than it was in the beginning of the last century. Indeed, the fastest growing segment of our population is the 85 years and older crowd! There have been tremendous advances made in this century. We can stay younger longer. There are things we can do, daily routines we can change, to stay vital. And, of course, there are things we cannot change, that are a function of age, which both men and women must accept. Like Susan, we have to learn which is which—and how to use those things we *can* change for optimal results.

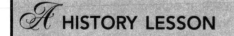

A HISTORY LESSON

Although you might wish to turn back the clock, you don't want to go too far back in time. You are very lucky to age in this century, not in ancient Rome, not in Victorian England, not even in the Roaring Twenties. Imagine . . .

Living to the ripe old age of 18—if a Tyrannosaurus Rex didn't get you in prehistoric America.

Seeing your husband, your "master" facing his first ancient Roman Senate race as a preteen—so he could have a full political career before he dies—at the average age of 22. (Forget about your political aspirations; you're busy being held captive at home in the villa.)

Praying that your father found a wonderful man for you to marry in the Gothic cathedral in your medieval realm—at the almost "too mature" age of 13.

Or even hoping that you'll live long enough to ride alongside your husband in one of those new-fangled cars displayed at the 1900 World's Fair—when living past 45 is considered a push.

Thanks to factors like the plague, polluted drinking water, and just plain ignorance, our ancestors didn't stand a chance—even if they chose not to fight in the Crusades or their wealth enabled them to live sequestered in country manors.

And women? True, they didn't have to put on their armor and fight infidels, but they were still not immune to the germs, the superstitions, and the pollution. Worse, even if they lived in a germfree, purified environment, they'd still have to contend with being considered inferior to men: second-class citizens at best, chattel or property at worst. Remember, women's rights didn't become a concept, or suffragette a word, until well into the 19th century.

But today the possibilities are endless for both men and women. Our life expectancy has exploded. In comparison to an average age of 47.3 in 1915, the U.S. Census Bureau has calculated that, today, women can easily live to 75.8 and beyond. In fact, centurions will no longer be rarities, people celebrated on television as their birthdays approach. By the year 2004, there will be 140,000 of us over 100 years old! Inroads in medicine and science, combined with a public that is more informed and more enlightened, ensure not only that we can live long, healthy lives—but live these years well.

That doesn't mean, however, that you can spend your life eating fatty foods, sprawled on the couch, or hanging out in smoky bars. Consider the fact that, thanks to habitual smoking and *schnapps*, the average life span in Russia is only 60.

In other words, we can live longer and healthier—as long as we change certain habits, certain mindsets, and adapt.

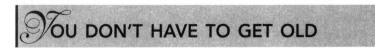

YOU DON'T HAVE TO GET OLD

Aging is not the same thing as getting older. True, the numbers continue to get higher, even if we start to ignore our birthdays. We can't turn back the clock. Nor can we ignore heredity, the genes that make us vulnerable to a particular disease, to some "weak link" in our family history. But we *can* help prevent a vulnerability from becoming a *fait accompli*. We can prevent further damage. We *can* successfully treat conditions and prevent them from becoming worse.

Our fate doesn't have to be etched in stone. Many illnesses are a result of lifestyle, not DNA. Heart disease, depression, digestive distress, hypertension, diabetes, chronic pain, and sexual dysfunction are only a few of the conditions that may be controlled with healthy habits and a positive mindset.

In short, a strong, solid optimistic emotional and mental attitude can keep us young—despite the passing years.

THE BABY BOOMER'S GUIDE TO WOMEN'S HEALTH

This book is all about staying young. Feeling optimistic and energetic. Joyful and healthy. It is for women like you and unlike you —everywhere across the globe. It is for all female "aging baby boomers" who have suddenly found themselves with an invitation to join the American Association of Retired Persons (AARP). It is for women who find themselves in the seemingly impossible position of growing old, a different "old" than the men in their lives: hormonally, sexually, and physically—with all the baggage they seem to carry when that first wrinkle appears, that menstrual cycle first becomes erratic. It will help women separate fact from fiction, discover what they can control in the aging process, and what must be accepted.

You can either spend these "golden years" desperate and anxious, like Susan in our example did, or you can flourish, feeling energized and content. This book will teach you how to make positive thinking a part of your life. It will help you discover how golden these years can really be. It will help you separate the myths from the realities, the functions of aging we cannot change and those we can do something about.

The first part of *The Baby Boomer's Guide to Women's Health* is all about the process of aging, the biological changes that occur in every woman. You will find in detail the changes that occur in your brain, your digestive tract, your bladder, your skin, and more, literally from the inside out. You'll also learn about important new theories that are being put forward on the subject of aging.

Using the metaphor of a house, the next section of this book helps you visualize the different areas of the your body and the specific conditions that can occur in each area—conditions that, although possible results of aging, *don't have to be.* You'll learn what to do about memory loss (the attic), hormone fluctuation (insulation), vision loss (windows), mobility problems (stairs), skin (the front yard), and more. In clear and compassionate terms, you'll be able to understand what causes a particular condition and how you can prevent it or stop it from getting worse. You'll find out what vitamins and minerals can help enhance your health and slow your particular condition—as well as what lifestyle changes you can implement right now to keep disease at bay. Like a house, with a little work, a little knowledge, your mind and body can stay firm, strong, and solid through the years.

In short, in this single volume you'll find everything you need to know about the aging process in women: what you can control and what you can't, and what you can do about making aging a relatively painless process. You'll learn to see yourself in a whole new light, a more hopeful and accepting light. You'll see that aging is not growing old. It is all about staying young.

Enjoy!

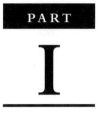

PART

I

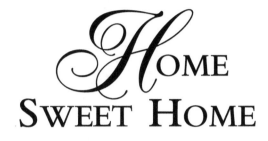

HOME
SWEET HOME

CHAPTER

1

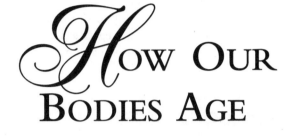

$\mathscr{H}$OW OUR BODIES AGE

Many more surprises concerning the aging process
are likely to be forthcoming. . . . The questions never end,
they just get more complex.
—Reubin Andres, MD
A participant in The Baltimore
Longitudinal Study of Aging

Myth: Our physical and mental capacities stay at the same level throughout our whole lives—until we become senior citizens.

Fact: The changes our bodies go through are dynamic; there is no set age when we might notice an ache when we walk, a need to turn the volume up.

Myth: Turn 65 and forget about it. It's all downhill with a capital "D"—for Dependency.

Fact: Eighty-seven percent of us who turn 65 are not only able to work and deal with everyday stress, but continue to live full and healthy lives.

Myth: Physical aging doesn't have to take place if we continue to stay active.

Fact: Startling as it seems, our physical abilities reach their peak *before we turn 21!* Throughout our adult lives, our abilities change—but so subtly that only gymnasts or professional athletes will notice the differences early on. Why don't we see the decline? *Because as a body ages, the mind gets finer-tuned; it compensates for any physical decline.*

Mention the word *aging* and everyone within earshot will have an opinion. And, as the above myths show, many of these opinions will be misguided and just plain negative. The truth is that aging, as with everything in life, has its good and bad elements.

THE GOOD STUFF

We can all make our own personal lists of the "bad" things about aging, things we have to accept in order to feel comfortable as the years pass. To help with handling the inevitable, we'll make jokes about our graying hair, our "senior moment" memory lapses, our sagging breasts and chins. They become material for birthday cards, stand up comic routines, and sit coms.

But what about the good? The qualities of aging that, like fine wine, *improve* in the golden years? Believe it or not, there are quite a few:

Experience counts for a lot. "The older we get, the wiser we become" is not just a cliché—it's the truth. The more we know, the more information we can use to better understand and perform. Our executive functions, those skills that help us focus, stay organized, and plan, become more sharply developed.

Maturity is a good thing. There's nothing more embarrassing than people not acting their age. Like the gray-haired, former cheerleader trying to keep her "school days" alive by nagging the "young 'uns" at every local game. The woman of a certain age who wears mini-skirts and blue nailpolish. The gum-popping, pot-bellied grandma trying to recapture "Dirty Dancing" on the dance floor. We feel embarrassed for these people. Far better to act our age, poised and graceful. And with this maturity, comes more than a "class act" persona. We'll be less impulsive—and exhibit better judgment. We'll be able to solve problems that used to panic us. We'll be more flexible. We'll have self-control, self-discipline, and a healthy perspective— in other words: maturity.

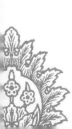

ONCE UPON A TIME

We're not the first people to ponder the process of aging. As long ago as ancient Greece, the physician Galen believed that aging was caused by such internal factors as bile and water which, over time, made us more susceptible to dryness and cold. In the Middle Ages scientist Roger Bacon felt that good hygiene could stop the wear and tear of the body. A century later, Charles Darwin applied aging to his "survival of the fittest" theory. He believed that we aged because our nervous system and muscles became apathetic; they responded to stimuli less and less.

Steady routines make for stress-free living. As we age the routines we follow become fine tuned; they are in place. Reading the paper in the morning is not only more enjoyable, but we browse through it more efficiently. Driving a car becomes second nature; we are better drivers in our 40s than in our roaring 20s. Going for a walk after dinner becomes a peaceful joy, not a chore we have to do to stay fit.

Stopping to smell the roses. The more we live life, the more we appreciate it. We count our blessings. We know how important our health is. The body has a great capacity to heal itself; we can live with only a single lung or kidney. But we cannot survive without our brain and our heart. As we age, we learn to appreciate our minds, our ability to move, our lives. And, as we exercise, as we eat right, as we keep a positive attitude, we know we're doing it for ourselves, for the *me,* for our physical and mental health. And it feels great!

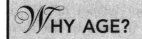 WHY AGE?

It's one thing to appreciate your age, to grow old with grace, but there's still the irony of "why." Yes, your executive functions are getting fine tuned. Your experience is paying off. You're more at peace with your life than ever before. But, let's face it, it would be nice to have all these plusses—and the body and face of a vivacious 20-year-old woman!

Aging, like taxes, is a fact of life. Here are some current theories that explain why:

"Oh, My Aging Genes" or the Genetic Cellular Theory

As you learned way back in biology, DNA is the stuff of life. Basically, it is protein that is set up in specific codes resembling a kind of twisting ladder within each and every one of your cells; these codes determine the color of your eyes, your bone structure, the amount of hair you'll have on your head at 20, 30, and 60. In other words, every bit of you—from the deepest recesses of your brain to the soles of your feet—is formed, developed, and sustained by the way the DNA in your cells is stacked up, or encoded.

A scientist in New Orleans has recently been able to isolate 14 genes that determine life span. Other studies have isolated a "death gene" that can shorten life. Still other studies have found a "clock mechanism" within our cells that determines how long a cell will function and replicate (i.e. reproduce) before it dies. All total, the current research suggests that there are possibly hundreds of genes within our bodies that predetermine how long we will live—in the same way that other genes control our hair color and height. The good news? As scientists continue to isolate "aging" genes, they can learn how to actually add proteins to our cells; they can change the code of a DNA strand. Instead of a "death" gene, we may have life!

"Blue Genes" or the DNA "Toxic-Shock" Theory

Cells are efficient entities. They can grow, divide, and replicate; building our bodies, hearts, and minds, from the inside out. When we react to stress, our cells reverberate within us. It is cells that send messages to and from the brain regarding a trauma we are feeling or perceiving. It is cells that create a sharp pain, a tear in the eye. And, located within each of our billions of cells, is DNA—which can also react to the shock of stress. In fact, there is one particular strand of DNA protein that exists specifically to help the cell respond and cope with stress. It's called *heated shock protein* (HSP). Scientists at the Gerontology Research Center in Baltimore, Maryland, have found that cells produce less and less HSP as we age. What does this mean? As we grow older, it is possible that we can cope less with stress, especially physical stress. And, because stress itself can make us feel old, lower HSP levels in our cells becomes a true paradox: the difficulties we have in dealing with stress generates even more stress. The best advice: Learn how to cope with stress in your everyday life. Maintain a healthy lifestyle. It will keep the emotional and physical shocks and stresses that age us at bay. (*See Chapter Five, Keeping Depression at Bay, as well as Part III of this book.*)

"Throw the Garbage Out Now!" or the Accumulation Damage Theory

Over time, waste begins to build up in a cell. Dark, globby, and seemingly invincible, this substance, called lipofuscin, eventually takes up so much room that cell function is impaired. The cell can get sluggish and eventually die.

Other "toxic" waste includes free radicals—oxygen-deprived molecules that are a byproduct of normal metabolism. Thanks to their craving for oxygen, these greedy free radicals combine quickly and easily with other more enriched molecules in the cell. The new chemical combinations that result from this union can damage cells and their DNA. Aging is accelerated.

But the body has a built-in defense against free radicals: antioxidants. In the best science fiction fashion, antioxidant enzymes, such as superoxide dismutase (SOD), and antioxidant vitamins, such as C and E, attack the free radicals floating around in a cell and neutralize them. Some of these enzymes "eat" the cell damage caused by free radicals and other toxins. Still others repair damaged protein. We don't even have to wait for the body's antioxidants to "kick in." We can add our own troops by routinely taking vitamin A, C, and E supplements—antioxidants all.

IT'S NEVER TOO LATE

At the age of 67, a woman named Emma Gatewood decided to take a hike. She ended up walking the entire length of the Appalachian Trail, from Maine to Georgia. She had such a good time that in her seventies she hiked the trail again—twice.

"I Have Seen the Enemy and It is Us" or the Immune System Decline Theory

Our immune system literally saves our lives, tirelessly seeking out alien viruses, bacteria, germs, and bacteria that have invaded our bodies. Once an alien is recognized, specialized cells called B-lymphocytes produce antibodies that ward off the aliens and render them harmless. Other cells called T-lymphocytes (T-cells) aggressively attack the foreigners, destroying them on impact. As we grow older, T-cells and antibodies lose some of their efficiency. They become sluggish; they cannot always recognize an alien from a "friend." Normal, healthy cells are destroyed by mistake; alien germs and viruses are able to permeate cells and mutate them—and their DNA.

Some scientists call this the "disease of aging." And it is true that the decline of the immune system can make us more susceptible to cancers, pneumonia, and other diseases. But there has been promising research done with DHEA (dehydroepiandrosterone) in Salt Lake City, Utah. A hormone produced by the body, DHEA, has been linked to the immune system and the aging process. We begin to produce less and less DHEA from age 30 on; when laboratory rats were given DHEA as a supplement their immune systems received a dramatic boost. However, don't run out and start taking DHEA just yet. Many more studies must be performed. But it's a promising beginning!

"My Biological Clock is Ticking" or the Hormonal Balance Theory

The nervous system (especially the hypothalamus in your brain) and the endocrine system (including the pancreas and the pituitary, thyroid, and adrenal glands) work in tandem to efficiently produce chemicals called hormones. These hormones, or chemicals, in turn, regulate our metabolism, our blood glucose levels, our body temperature, and our ability to cope with changes in the environment. And, as every woman knows, they also regulate our menstrual cycle and the onset of menopause. (Remember how your heart beat wildly, your face flushed, and your whole body "revved up" the last time your car skidded, your child leaned back in her chair, or you thought you were going to have a "hot flash" in front of the whole conference room? That's your neuro-endocrine system as its best, getting you ready for action.)

Unfortunately, the endocrine system begins to decline with age. Studies have found that the pancreas in older people, for example, does not release enough of the hormone insulin when a meal has been eaten. Insufficient amounts of insulin means that blood-sugar levels will rise—and adult-onset diabetes can occur.

Another example: As we know, estrogen production stops at menopause. When estrogen production stops, women age more rapidly and may become more susceptible to heart attacks; they may also experience sexual dysfunction. Hormonal Replacement Therapy (HRT) may protect against several problems related to aging. (*See Chapter Six.*) But what might not be common knowledge is that a link exists between estrogen and the hypothalamus. The hypothalamus, deep within the brain, tells the pituitary gland to produce estrogen; it must also tell the gland to stop. What does this mean? *That a biological clock must reside in the hypothalamus, a clock that regulates aging.* Identify this timepiece and who knows? Like any good watch, it may be able to be repaired and restored—for many years.

Welcome to the world of aging. Yes, there are some harsh and complicated truths, but they are countered by endless possibilities. The future is not yet here.

2

*M*IRROR, MIRROR ON THE WALL: VISIBLE AGING

The secret of staying young is to live honestly,
eat slowly, and lie about your age.
—Lucille Ball

- Danielle cringed whenever she looked in the mirror. She didn't see her startlingly pretty green eyes. She didn't see her beautiful, thick red hair. As far as she was concerned, all the mirror reflected back were the crow's feet around her eyes, her puffy eyelids, her fuller chin. Forget the hair, the eyes, the lovely smile. Danielle didn't see any of them.
- Miriam knew she was losing her hair. But instead of accepting the fact that her thick, shoulder-length hair was a thing of the past, she tried to disguise its new wispiness with hats and extensions and, every once in a while, a wig. Unfortunately, Miriam was fooling no one but herself. She didn't look attractive; she didn't look young. In fact, her attempts to keep her long hair made her look even older than she was.

- "What?" Ginny seemed to always ask. "What did you say?" Sometimes she became so tired of asking people to repeat themselves that she ignored the fact that she couldn't hear. She missed conversations. Plays. Movies. A hearing aid would have taken care of the problem, but Ginny refused to get fitted for one. It would mean that she was getting old.

- Joan's feet were killing her. She was athletic, trim; she even had smooth, unlined skin. Joan never thought of herself as "old." She worked hard at keeping healthy. But, despite all her good work, her doctor recently diagnosed her with gout. Gout! Joan always thought of gout as a disease that only fat, dissolute, slovenly people got—like Henry VIII in his old age. Yet here Joan was, not even 60, with such pain in her feet that she couldn't even do her morning jog. It was just as well. Joan was so depressed about her condition that she didn't feel like exercising ever again.

These four women are not alone. As we've already mentioned, America is home to 31 million aging baby boomers—and counting. At one time or another, most of these millions and millions of people, your friends, your families, your co-workers, even your neighborhood deli owner or your dry cleaner clerk—all of them (and all of us)—have looked in the mirror and noticed a line here, a sagging chin there. All of us have looked aging in the face and come up short.

But as much as the aging process is a fact of life, it doesn't have to engulf us. Knowing the facts about aging—what we can change and what we can't—can make all the difference between growing old gracefully and aging full of despair. Education can help us understand how we'll change as we get old. With fewer surprises, we may become more accepting, and, most important of all, less fearful. To that end, let's talk about some of the visible signs of aging:

More Than Skin Deep: Aging and Your Skin

Gravity, the same force that keeps you firmly planted to terra firma, is unfortunately responsible for your skin to start sagging. By the time you've reached your fifties, gravity has pushed two-thirds of your face down—which is why your chin, cheekbones, nose, and mouth may look droopy.

Lines are a different story. Aging is responsible for some of your crow's feet and wrinkles; years of wear, frowns, laughter, and squinting do etch their marks on your skin. But most of the lines and brown age spots you hate to see in the mirror come from sun damage you did to your skin—in your twenties! Eighty percent of your lines, wrinkles, and age spots are due to this photoaging.

But the worst by-product of our sunbathing youth, by far, is skin cancer. Basal cell carcinomas are the most common form; these skin cancers don't usually spread to other organs. Squamous cell carcinomas are more serious because they do spread to other parts of your body. Malignant melanomas are extremely dangerous and can be fatal. The good news is that skin cancer can be easily treated—if caught early enough. If you notice a change in the shape and color of a mole, see your doctor immediately. Make sure you get a "skin check" by your family physician once a year. If that's not possible, have your spouse or a friend check those areas you cannot see—like the center of your back where most melanomas occur in men.

As you reach your fifties, collagen, the elastic, connective fiber in the skin that makes it supple and resilient, begins to decrease. (This is why so many skin products for "mature-skinned women" are labeled collagen-enriched). Given the fact that your skin also loses water as you age, it's easy to see why you have more pronounced wrinkles and lines.

Dry skin is another "joy" of aging. It affects approximately 85% of adults because, as we age, we don't sweat as much and our oil

THE OLDER BLUSH

Just when you think it's safe to pass your pimple medicine to your teenager, adult acne rears its ugly head. The hormonal changes in later life can produce adult acne, especially rosacea, rosy, pimply blotches around your nose and on your cheeks. The "blush" comes from minute broken blood vessels and it can be made worse by too much alcohol, chocolate, spicy foods, or caffeine. Antibiotics can control rosacea, and lasers can eliminate its uneven "glow."

glands produce fewer hormones. To help avoid dry, itchy, irritated skin, use a humidifier when indoors; take showers instead of hot, lingering baths; and apply antiperspirants and perfumes lightly.

You can find out more about your skin and how it ages from:

The American Academy of Dermatology
930 North Meacham Road
Schaumburg, IL 606173-4965
1-847-330-0230
www.aad.org

The Skin Cancer Foundation
245 Fifth Avenue, Suite 2402
New York, NY 10016
1-800-SKIN-490
www.skincancer.org

Hair Today, Gone Tomorrow: Aging and Your Hair

Whether you call it irony, a cruel twist of fate, or genetic coding, the facts stay the same: as we age, our hair gets thinner where we want it—and thicker where we don't. The rate of hair growth on the head diminishes after the age of 65; individual strands grow in less thick. Conversely, although the reason is not clear, men usually get longer, darker, thicker hair growth in their ears, eyebrows, noses, and on their backs. Women usually sprout their "new" hair on their lips and chins.

Other "hairy" traits include:

• You can thank your genes for male pattern baldness, which occurs in 75% of women. It starts in a circle at the top of the head and moves outward. The good news is that it is rarely as severe in women as it is in men.
• Hair begins to turn gray after the age of 40 when your hair color starts to lose its pigment. Both hormonal changes and heredity play a role.

Growing Pains: Aging and Your Height

The same force that affects your face does a number on your body: gravity. Years of physical pressure literally "push" your body toward earth. Muscles weaken and, as a result of the reduction of an amino acid called creatinine (it helps bones stay toned and supple), we lose some of that lean muscle mass we exercised to get. Water loss in the disks between the bones of your spine makes your skeletal structure compress. Bones become more brittle and posture becomes more stooped. You actually begin to shrink. Women can lose as much as two inches because of water loss in the disks of the spine and calcium loss (and the subsequent risk of osteoporosis) after menopause.

At the same time that your frame becomes more fragile and stooped, cartilage, the connective fiber found in bone, builds up. This excess cartilage makes your nose, ears, and even the width of your feet larger. Features can become so prominent that you may look as if you are "all" nose or ears.

If you have questions about your bones, contact:

The National Institute of Arthritis and Musculoskeletal and Skin Diseases (NIAMS) Clearinghouse
1 AMS Circle
Bethesda, MD 20892-3675
(301) 495-4484
www.nih.gov/NIAMS

Amidst this bone-chilling information, there is hope—and its name is exercise. Research has shown that exercise, especially strength-training with weights, can help reduce the loss of lean muscle mass as well as keep bones strong. Go for it!

Weighty Issues: Aging and Your Weight

Here's another reason to exercise: weight maintenance. Unfortunately, as your lean muscle mass starts to weaken, your adipose tissue, or fat cells, increases. Studies show that this excess fat is a result of a decrease in water and potassium (a by-product of aging) within your body. Muscles need these elements; without proper amounts of water and potassium the food you eat turns not to muscle—but fat. Our metabolism slows; energy drops. In fact, even after the age of 20, we need to keep revved up; our resting metabolism, or basal metabolism, drops 10% every ten years!

Another reason for weight gain is lack of activity. You might have been a couch potato in your youth, but, when metabolism slows, that same sedentary lifestyle can pack on the calories. "Middle-age spread" is not a cliché; your body, particularly in the waist and chest, gets flabby. But a sagging, aging body doesn't have

to be your destiny. You have to defy the great "slow down" myth of aging. Instead, get active. Move. Start an exercise class. The more you move your body, the more calories you'll burn and the less food will be stored as fat.

Another reason to move? As you approach old age, the weight gain pendulum turns back. You will actually lose weight, but not in a positive way. Muscle weakness and deterioration can make you too thin. Exercise can help counteract the wear and tear of time by making your bones and muscles strong.

Say It Again: Aging and Your Voice

Thirteen-year-old boys are not the only ones whose voices change. As women age, their vocal cords become stiffer and begin to vibrate more quickly; their tone of voice may become two to three notes higher on the musical scale.

You also may find your voice quavering, similar to the "cracking" pitch young boys experience. This tremor in your voice may be accompanied by a tremor in your hands and a slight shaking of your head. This condition is called an "essential" or "senile tremor" and is a result of a slight loss of control over your vocal cords and neuromuscular system. It does not mean you are senile!

Say Cheese!: Aging and Your Teeth, Gums, and Mouth

Some people think that, as adults, they can keep away from the dentist. Like avoiding broccoli and brussels sprouts, they feel they can avoid the hated drill, the poking and prodding. But just as your parents knew that it was good for you to eat your vegetables, they were also wise in the ways of the 6-month dental checkup. Without a winning smile, you'll feel—and look—older than your years!

The most common tooth problem for adults over the age of 35 is periodontal (gum) disease. Three out of every 4 adults have had it at least once in their lives. Plaque, a sticky, yellowish substance made of bacteria from the proteins and sugars we eat, and tartar, which is dead, calcified plaque, find a home on our teeth, at our gumline, and sometimes beneath it in our gum tissue. Without professional cleaning by a dental professional, the bacteria in plaque and tartar build up, creating inflamed, bleeding gums (gingivitis); mouth pain; and bad breath. Gums begin to recede, leaving roots exposed to bacteria and tooth decay. (Receding gum lines also make teeth more sensitive to hot and cold, although this can also be a sign of root problems.) Eventually, the bacteria reach the tissue that supports your teeth. Roots become infected, teeth become loose, and, without root canal surgery, your teeth may simply fall out. But tooth loss—and resulting dentures—can be avoided simply by taking regular care of your gums. This means seeing your dentist on a regular basis—and eating your vegetables. (Good nutrition helps maintain healthy teeth.)

Another dental problem you might experience as you age is yellowing teeth. The visible layer of your teeth is covered in enamel, a porous, crystallized substance. Everyday wear and tear on your teeth can cause cracks and chips—which attract food stains. Add years of coffee or tea-drinking or smoking and it's no surprise that your teeth are no longer pearly white.

Dry mouth, or xerostomia, is another common problem as you age. It can affect the way you eat, speak, swallow, and taste. Medical professionals used to believe it was unavoidable as you age, as inevitable as wrinkles and gray hair. No more. Today we know that dry mouth can be caused by any one of more than over 400 medications! These include antihypertensives, diuretics, antihistamines, antidepressants, decongestants, and painkillers. Left to its own devices, dry mouth can cause further tooth decay. Without enough saliva to "wash away" food particles and debris, bacteria thrives. Excess plaque can eventually rule and, excuse the pun, wear a brand new crown.

As we age, restorations often become problematic. Fillings, crowns, and other previous dental work all become worn down over the years; they might need to be restored or replaced. Silver

THE RED FLAG

Bleeding gums are not just a sign of periodontal disease. If your gums bleed, it might mean vitamin deficiencies, diabetes, or, in rare cases, blood disorders. It can also be a side effect of hormone therapy or the use of anticoagulants such as Coumadin®. The best way to solve your "bleeding gums" mystery? See your dentist as soon as possible.

amalgam fillings can last up to 15 years; plastic tooth-colored fillings can last between 5 and 8 years; gold inlays can last up to 20 years; and porcelain, ceramic, and metal crowns and inlays can last up to 15 years.

Dentures require the same care as your "real" teeth. Poor dental hygiene and nutrition can create yellowing, periodontal disease, and bad breath. Brush your dentures, both partials and full, every day. Place them overnight in a cleaning solution designed specifically for dentures. Rinse your mouth with warm, salty water in the morning and after you eat. And, like new shoes, remember that your dentures take time to "wear in." Avoid sticky, hard food in the beginning. Cut food into small pieces. Chew slowly on the sides of your mouth, not in front. If you have problems adjusting to your dentures after a few weeks, see your dentist. They might not have been properly fitted.

Poor teeth, painful gums, and bad breath can hinder your social life; it can hurt your quality of life and make you feel older than you really are. But it doesn't have to be this way. Proper daily cleaning of your teeth or dentures can help prevent problems from taking root. Cosmetic bleaching can make yellow teeth white again. Cosmetic dentistry, including almost-invisible orthodontic braces, tooth bonding to smooth out color, and veneers placed over your teeth to change their shape, color, and texture can all go far in bringing a dazzle back to your smile. Find out more about your teeth, gums, and mouth from the:

National Institute of Dental Research
31 Center Drive/Building 31, Room 2C35
Bethesda, MD 20892-2290
(301) 496-4261
www.nidr.nih.gov

National Oral Health Information Clearinghouse
1 NOHIC Way
Bethesda, MD 20892-3500
(301) 402-7364
www.aerie.com/NOHIC

American Dental Association
211 East Chicago Avenue
Chicago, IL 60611
(800) 621-8099
www.ada.org

Step Lively: Aging and Your Feet

You can't change everything about your feet. Age is going to wear down your feet, the skin, ligaments, tendons, muscles, and even the padding at the balls of our feet and the heels. Your feet will lose some of their "bounce." Muscles will lose some of their elasticity and bones will lose some density.

But there are some "footfalls" you can control. Cramps in your feet. Pain when you walk. Bulging bunions and corns. These seemingly small irritations can make you feel and act old. They can sabotage your quality of life. But you don't have to necessarily "foot this bill."

Many of your foot problems started a long time ago. Years of wearing high heels, for example, can narrow your toe cage, squashing tender feet together and creating hammertoes, bunions, and other musculoskeletal deformities. Even worse, the Achilles' heel tendon in the back of your foot, from your ankle to your heel, can become foreshortened. This will make it painful to walk even when you fling off your high heels. (There's something to be said for wearing tennis shoes!)

Obesity can also affect your foot health. If you have been overweight for many years, your body's pounding against your feet as you walk will take its toll, most likely in painful spurs, or calcium deposits, on the bones of your feet, especially at your heels.

Another "heel": dry skin. The same reduced oil (sebaceous) gland production that affects your face as you age, also affects your feet—especially your heels. Dry, flaky skin can itch and burn; it can create cracks and fissures. Keep your feet moist by taking cooler showers in winter, applying moisturizer twice a day, and exfoliating the flakes with a pumice stone.

Exfoliation, however, will only go so far for corns and calluses. Because you lose some of the fat at the ball of your feet as you age, your tootsies get an extra pounding as you walk and go about your day. This extra pressure creates a protective layer of thick skin at the bony prominences at the sides of your toes and feet. Although this thick skin helps prevent cuts and bone damage, it can compress the nerves in your foot—which causes pain. Corns are just like calluses, but you'll usually find them at the tops of your toes; and they'll be more defined in shape. A podiatrist can remove corns and calluses; to prevent their reoccurrence, wear soft, comfortable shoes that fit.

Medical conditions such as diabetes can also affect your feet. Diabetes can impede circulation—sometimes literally stopping blood flow to your toes. (*See Chapter Six for a complete description of this disease.*)

Ingrown toenails are another painful foot problem. Contrary to popular opinion, they are not caused by cutting your nails improperly. Rather, the shape of your nail and your toe dictate whether or not you'll have an ingrown nail, usually on your big toe. Shoes that are too tight can exacerbate the problem. A podiatrist can remove the part of the nail that is pushing into your flesh. If necessary, the nail can be cauterized so it will stop growing.

Nail fungus is another joy of aging feet. Over the years, especially if you wear tight shoes, parts of your toenails, especially the big and little toes, can develop minute fissures, which allows fungus to invade the nail. Eventually, the fungus changes the nail, creating brittleness, changes in color, and thickening—which, in turn, makes trimming the nails difficult and painful. Fungus is more of an embarrassment than a medical threat. But a reluctance to take off your shoes and socks can make anyone feel uncomfortable. Avoid those negative feelings with antifungal medications; your doctor may even prescribe one of the new, effective oral medications. (Athlete's foot is also a fungus, but it occurs between the toes and on the soles. It is common among people of all ages and can usually be treated with over-the-counter powders and creams.)

Another factor of aging has nothing to do with the actual intrinsic nature of your feet and toes. It has to do with flexibility. As you get older, you might not be able to care for your feet as well as you once did. Perhaps you can't bend over to cut your nails. Your strength is off. Perhaps you can't maintain your balance when you try to wash your feet in the shower. Whatever the reason, negligence can create the above problems as easily as too-tight shoes. The best solution? A professional pedicure or, if that's not possible, a trim and a soak by a caregiver. Find more information by contacting the:

American Podiatric Medical Association
9312 Old Georgetown Road
Bethesda, MD 20814
(301) 571-9200
www.apma.org

IN GOOD COMPANY

Some people call it the disease of excess. Too much good living. Too much rich food and drink. Others call it genetic, a twist of fate. Whatever its real root, one thing is certain: Gout can cause terrible pain, especially in your big toes. It occurs when your body has trouble removing uric acid, a waste product of the amino acid purine (found in red meat, organ meat, poultry, beer, certain types of fish, cheese, and wine). The buildup of uric acid forms painful needle-like crystals in your toe. Your immune system then sends out its force of phagocytes, the cells that protect our body from germs, bacteria, and foreign debris. As the phagocytes dutifully break up the crystals, they ironically create pain-pounding inflammation. The result is gout, a scourge that hit the likes of Henry VIII and Ben Franklin.

A diet free of fatty meats and alcohol can help reduce the buildup of uric acid. Anti-inflammatory medications, such as Indomethacin, can help reduce the pain. Drugs such as allopurinol help prevent the body from producing uric acid and, taken daily as a preventative measure, can stop gout from recurring.

The Eyes Have It: Aging and Your Eyes

One of the most difficult by-products of aging we all have to accept is vision change. But change doesn't have to be bad. Yes, your eyes are going to weaken, but many women continue to have good vision in their 80s! If you can recognize the changes that occur in your eyes, you can do damage control:

- *Avoid eyestrain.* You might find it more difficult to see in dim light as you age. Don't pretend there's nothing wrong. Add some lights at your desk, near your easy chair, where you eat dinner. Put extra watts in wall fixtures, on stairwells, and you can help prevent an accident due to weak eyes.
- *Be kind to your "reading" eyes.* Presbyopia is a common condition in people over 40; it's a type of far-sightedness that's a

normal part of the aging process. You'll know if you have presbyopia if you need to keep menus and books at arm's length in order to read them, if the small print looks blurry, if your eyes get tired while reading, doing needlepoint, or performing close work. You can easily take control of presbyopia with reading glasses prescribed by your ophthalmologist. You can also go to your local drugstore and try a pair of off-the-shelf "readers."

- *Keep your eyes moist.* Dry eyes are a common complaint as people age. Tears come from the lacrimal glands located inside your eyelids. As you age, these glands can decrease their production of tears, and the composition of your tears can change. Dry eyes, with its symptoms of irritation, burning, itching, and sometimes loss of vision, is the result. You can keep dry eyes in check by using over-the-counter artificial teardrops and by keeping a humidifier on in your office and at home.

- *Protect your eyes from the environment.* You wear (hopefully!) sunblock when you're out in the sun to protect your body, but what about your eyes? They can get sunburned, too. (Too much sun as a teenager can increase the risk of cataracts and macular degeneration as you age.) Always wear sunglasses or a wide-brimmed hat when you are outside. Not only will sunglasses protect your eyes from a bright sun, but they can help prevent tearing due to too much wind or extreme temperature.

- *Schedule regular eye exams*—every year. Many of the medical conditions associated with age can be treated successfully—if caught early enough. By dilating your eyes and testing them, an ophthalmologist can catch such conditions as retinal detachment (one of the reasons for seeing "floaters"), glaucoma (a buildup of pressure inside the eye), macular degeneration (a loss of sharp vision), and cataracts (cloudiness in the lens of the eye). Specific medications and surgery, on an outpatient basis, can help most of these conditions before too much vision is lost. (*See Chapter Nine for details on these conditions and other age-related vision problems.*)

- *Treat the rest of your body well.* Having a physical exam on a regular basis is not only crucial to maintaining good health, but it can also help detect diseases that can cause eye problems. A simple blood test can determine if you have diabetes, which causes the small blood vessels in your retina to malfunction. The result? Diabetic retinopathy . . . and blindness.

Yes, you can have more eye problems now that you've gotten older. But they can be treated—and prevented—with a little foresight. Remember, hindsight is always 20/20! For more information, contact:

The National Eye Institute
2020 Vision Place
Bethesda, MD 20892-3655
(301) 496-5248
www.nei.nih.gov

The American Foundation for the Blind
11 Penn Plaza, Suite 300
New York, NY 10001
(800) 232-5463
www.afb.org

The American Optometric Association
243 North Lindbergh Boulevard
St. Louis, MO 63141
(314) 991-4100
www.aoanet.org

What Did You Say?: Aging and Your Hearing

Hearing loss is one of the most common—and most noticeable—characteristics of growing old. Hair cells in the inner ear, responsible for hearing, are lost, affecting the way we hear sound frequencies and speech discriminations. Exposure to loud noises, over time, erodes your ability to hear. You are not alone. Approximately one-third of all Americans over age 65 have some kind of hearing problem. By 85, the number increases to one-half. The hearing loss can be as simple as missing some lines of dialogue at a play or not hearing the phone—or as complex as total deafness.

Some age-related conditions of the ear include:

• *Presbycusis.* Almost everyone over the age of 65 will have this hearing disorder—the very gradual loss of hearing due to changes in the inner ear. You might not be able to hear people speaking clearly, and you will be more irritated by loud noises. Like the appearance of gray hair, the change is slow, over time, and the rate of change is different for everyone.

- *Tinnitus.* Ringing in the ear. It's another common hearing ailment that results from obstruction in the ear canal (possibly by wax), middle ear abnormalties, or taking certain medication, such as an excessive amount of aspirin. Tinnitus can also signal an inner ear or a nerve disorder, however, and should be checked by your doctor. The truth is, most of the time, the cause cannot be identified. Fortunately, tinnitus is rarely more than a nuisance.

- *Conductive and sensorineural hearing loss.* Medication, high blood pressure, a stroke, a tumor, head injury, poor circulation, ear wax build-up, middle-ear infection, even a common cold—these can all create problems in your ear. In a conductive hearing loss, sounds are blocked from entering the inner ear. Sensorineural hearing loss is more serious; it means that damage has occurred to the hair cells in the inner ear or to the hearing nerve. (*Read about hearing disorders in depth in Chapter Ten.*)

Hearing loss does not have to mean the end of the world. Today, hearing aids, which work by amplifying sound, are excellent; there are hearing aids to fit every need and budget. You can get a hearing aid that can barely be detected in your ear; you can get one that adjusts to frequency and environment. Implantable hearing aids are presently being investigated in Europe and in the United States. (Cochlear implants are also available for certain patients with specific types of severe to profound sensorineural hearing loss and in instances where a hearing aid is not helpful.) If you believe you have a hearing problem, don't wait until it gets worse. See your doctor now—and hear what he has to say! For more information, you can contact the:

**American Academy of Otolaryngology—Head
and Neck Surgery, Inc.**
One Prince Street
Alexandria, VA 22314
(703) 836-4444
(703) 519-1585 (TTY)
www.entnet.org

American Speech Language Hearing Association
10801 Rockville Pike/Dept. AP
Rockville, MD 20852
(800) 638-8255 (Voice/TTY)

We've now finished with the outside of our "house," the paint, the shingles, the lawn—all the signs of aging that we can see. It's time now to investigate the interior, for the signs of aging we cannot see from the outside.

CHAPTER

3

AGING
WE CAN'T SEE

You don't stop laughing because you grow old;
you grow old because you stop laughing.
—Anonymous

Close your eyes and, in your mind, go back in time, to when you were a child. Picture yourself greeting your grandparents, hugging them and pulling them by the arm into the house. You remember your mother shouting, "Don't pull. Walk slowly! Grandma can't move as fast as you can." You remember their grunts as they settled on the sofa, the difficulty they had in getting up. The little hair your grandfather had was stone gray; you loved staring at his shiny pate. They had so many wrinkles you could barely see their eyes. To your eyes, these people were old, as old as time, with their stomach problems, their bulky bodies, their lack of energy. And of course they were old . . . they had to be at least 50!

Absurd, isn't it, to think of 50 as ancient. Perhaps it was more the norm "to look your age" 40 or 60 years ago; today those norms have not only gone out the window. We know more—and do more—to prevent aging than any generation before us. We know that the "50" of our grandparents is a far cry from the "50" of today. But attitudes still die hard. Preconceived notions have a way of sticking.

How do you rate on the "aging image" scale? Take this brief quiz and see how many questions you answer correctly. The results may surprise you.

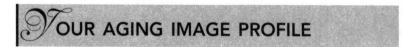

YOUR AGING IMAGE PROFILE

Read these statements and mark each one true or false:

1. If one of your parents has Alzheimer's disease, the chances are good that you too will eventually get it.
2. The fear of falling goes hand in hand with getting old—and with good reason.
3. Everyone gets "senior moments," lapses in memory that become more and more frequent as you get older.
4. Incontinence is a fact of life for "old folks."
5. Sexual desire is a thing of the past once you hit 60.
6. People get "crotchety" in their old age. Personalities change —for the worse.
7. You sleep less in old age because you need less sleep.
8. Depression is rampant among seniors.
9. It doesn't make sense to get regular checkups past the age of 65. If your doctor finds something, like heart disease or cancer, there's nothing she can do about it. You're too old.
10. The older you get, the more medication you can expect to take.

See the answers below to see how you did:

1. **False.** Although scientists have discovered a gene that may cause Alzheimer's disease in the small number of families who already have a high incidence rate, most people do not inher-it the gene. Alzheimer's is not cast in stone, or, in this case, genetic code.
2. **True.** Falls in the elderly are one of the leading reasons for disability. It is the most common cause of injury in people over 65. As vision and hearing deteriorate, perception becomes clouded. Dizziness and numbness in the feet can lead to poor balance. Stiff joints can affect your ability to

respond to obstacles. You can avoid pitfalls by getting regular checkups and making your house fall-proof. Remove stray wires and loose carpets. Keep floors clean without slippery wax. "Light up your world" with high wattage bulbs and night-lights. See if your local rehabilitation hospital has a fall-prevention program.

3. **False.** "Senior moments" can happen to thirtysomethings, generation Xers, even teens. Yes, memory lapses can be a symptom of Alzheimer's disease, but they can also be the result of having too much to do, depression, overwhelming stress, or even a side effect of a medication you are taking.

4. **False**. While it's true that the muscles that work your bladder weaken over time, incontinence does not have to be the end result. Muscles can be strengthened through exercise; your bladder can be controlled with various medications. *(See Chapter Twelve.)* Urinary incontinence is not an illness that stands alone; it is a symptom resulting from such conditions as head injury, stroke, spinal cord injury, urinary infections, even pregnancy. In short, it can occur to anyone—at any age. Check with your doctor or rehabilitation hospital to see if you would benefit from a continence program.

5. **False.** Just ask any senior! The loss of sexual desire is more the function of psychological and physical ailments. Because women in their 60s might show signs of depression or menopause, we tend to lump the symptoms all together and call it a "lack of desire"—when nothing could be further from the truth. In reality, as a survey conducted by the National Council on the Aging discovered, many Americans over 60 are interested in sex—and approximately one-half of those interviewed enjoy sex with a partner at least once a month. For many women, the main problem is the lack of a partner—not the lack of desire. *(See Chapter Eleven for more information on sexual matters.)*

6. **False.** There's an old expression: "You don't change as you age. You become more so." In other words, except for personality changes resulting from dementia, the way you laugh, the way you speak, the essence of you, the "soul" that makes you unique, stays with you for life. Even better: Many seniors "mellow out" as working, raising a family, and making a mark are no longer the central focuses of their lives.

7. **False.** It's not the amount of sleep that changes as you age, but the quality. Studies show that the older you are, the more your sleep is "broken up." You tend to be more restless at night; you'll take more naps during the day. You also might need to relieve yourself more frequently as you age, the result of a weakened bladder or medication.

8. **False.** Depression affects over 25% of all Americans—of all ages. Although it can be a symptom of the hormonal changes occurring in later life, depression is not necessarily age-related: stress, trauma, and transitions occur throughout life. The good news is that a wide variety of medications and therapies are available today to treat depression. (*See Chapter Five for more details.*)

9. **False.** Fatalistic thinking can become a self-fulfilling prophecy. If you believe that a condition is hopeless, it will be. Because you won't do the things you need to do in order to halt the process. The reality is that certain diseases, such as heart disease or cancer, are more common in people over 65. But that just means you need to be more vigilant. Instead of canceling your physical exams, you should increase them. Many forms of cancer can be beaten—if caught early enough.

10. **True.** Over 25% of all medications are prescribed for senior citizens. Conditions that take years to build up, such as high cholesterol, hypertension, osteoporosis, arthritis, and diabetes, may become serious enough to warrant medications as we age. But because there are so many different medications on the market, your doctor can find the right one for you—and keep most problems in check. Make sure you tell her about all the medications you are taking, from over-the-counter pain relievers to vitamins. Many people feel too embarrassed to tell their doctor about the herbs, supplements, and vitamins and minerals they are taking. There are adverse side-effects (contraindications) with certain combinations of pills that you are not aware of. Don't sit back and put up with side effects from your medicines. Ask your doctor to work with you on changing your medication.

By taking the time to take your "aging image" profile, you've learned a little more about your body, mind, and the aging process. Hopefully, you've also put some erroneous myths to rest.

Aging is a state of mind, as this profile points out—but only up to a point. There are certain things we cannot control, certain things that will change as we grow old. We've already explored the "surface" issues, the exterior of your "house," your skin, eyes, ears, and more, in the previous chapter. Now it's time to open the door and go inside, to the bones and muscles, nerves and arteries, organs and glands, that have grown up with you—and see what to expect in your 50s and beyond.

"A Bone to Pick" or Bone Loss and Shrinking Muscle

You can run, but you can't hide. As you age your muscles won't let you go as fast as you once did. You can push and push, exercise hours every day, but the fact is that your muscles will lose some of their tone and strength with age. How much? That depends on your total body weight and how fit you have been your whole life. (Another reason why a regular exercise routine and a nutritious diet are so important.) Research bears this out. There is a drop in potassium levels as people age. Because muscle composition has a higher potassium level than adipose tissue (read: fat cells!), this decrease is directly translated into less muscle mass and more body fat.

In old age muscles don't grow. Instead of bulging, muscle fiber slowly converts to connective tissue, which leads to stiffer, sore

---

TENNIS, ANYONE?

By the time you are 25, your muscles have reached their peak. From then on, you'll lose about 4% of muscle mass every ten years until you reach 50—when the loss accelerates to 10%!

To make matters more compromising, our cells also become less efficient after 50. They can't utilize oxygen as well—which translates into diminished endurance. Add brittle bones, which lessen our flexibility, and inner ear erosion, which affects our coordination, and a walk in the park can feel like a triathlon. The solution? Start exercising. Now. The more active you are now, no matter what your age, the less your body will be "stung" by the age bug.

muscles after physical exertion—and, unfortunately, fat. Your body becomes softer, rounder, and, at the same time, less flexible. It becomes more difficult to maintain a firm handgrip, to use your knees. Studies show that, on average, there is a 20% decrease in muscle power after the age of 70.

Your bones and your joints, too, feel the effects of age. You might experience more backaches in later life simply because of wear and tear on your spine and the soft-tissue, cushioning disks between each bony vertebra of your spine.

Then there are the "itises," a phrase coined in a *Newsweek* article, which include arthritis, tendinitis, and bursitis. All can be caused by wear and tear; it's all a question of where. In arthritis, it's the cartilage (the smooth shiny substance on the surface of your joints) that breaks down over time. Osteoarthritis, the official name for this type of arthritis, affects about 16 million Americans, many of them in old age. It hits hardest in the joints of your fingers, your hips, knees, and lower back.

Tendinitis comes from too much repetitive action over too much time. The tendons, which ensure muscles adhere to bones, become swollen and inflamed. What areas are most susceptible? Shoulder cuffs and elbows. ("Tennis elbows" don't need a racquet to be felt.) Golfers, hockey players, swimmers, volleyball enthusiasts—women in all these fields, over time, can develop tendinitis.

Believe it or not, bursitis is not a name simply conjured up from thin air. It is derived from the more than 150 bursae in our body that can become inflamed over time. What are bursae? They are the fluid-filled pads, the "fluffy pillows" of our bodies, that make ligaments, tendons, and bones all come together comfortably at a joint. Strain, overuse, and ordinary wear and tear over the years can produce inflammation in these bursae, particularly in the shoulders, hips, knees, and elbows. This inflammation, in turn, results in an outpouring of excess fluid in the bursae—which puts pressure on the surrounding tissue. The ultimate result? Chronic pain.

Wear and tear aren't the only villains in town. Muscle, balance, and coordination damage from stroke and other conditions affecting the nervous system can be just as harmful—and show their potency faster than age's erosion—by causing flaccid muscles, paralysis, and unsteady gaits.

Your autoimmune system is also, excuse the pun, not immune to bone and muscle damage. Rheumatoid arthritis (RA), unlike its "wear and tear" arthritic cousin, is a disease of the autoimmune system; it is caused by an inflammation of these same joints. RA can be the result of your long-ago encoded genes or a viral infection—worsened by stress or illness.

Osteoporosis, the buzzword for any woman over 50, is the result of age, yes, but not overuse. In fact, exercise can stave off its worst symptoms: fragility, bone fractures, and disfigurement. Although osteoporosis occurs slowly, over a long time, it usually isn't noticed until after menopause—when the drop in estrogen accelerates the symptoms. (*See Chapter Eight to find out all the details on osteoporosis.*)

If you have any signs of bone and muscle aging, you might find some of these organizations helpful:

The National Osteoporosis Foundation
1150 17th Street, NW, Suite 602
Washington, DC 20036-2226
(800) 223-9994
(202) 223-2226
www.nof.org

The Arthritis Foundation
1330 West Peachtree Street
Atlanta, GA 30309
(404) 872-7100
http://www.arthritis.org

"Learned by Heart" or Cardiovascular Aging

It's time for some good news, and it comes from the heart. Research has found that the heart actually compensates for age, adjusting to the ups and downs of life by growing thick walls. This "thicker skin" is most noticeable in the left ventricle, the "king" of the heart's four heart-pumping chambers, which works the hardest to get your blood moving throughout your system. These thick walls help the blood move more efficiently through less flexible, aging arteries.

Changes also occur in the mitral valve. This is the gateway between the all-important left ventricle and the chamber directly above it: the left atrium. Blood from the left atrium rushes into the left ventricle through this valve in two waves; the first wave is called *action potential*; the second is called a *late surge*. As you age, it takes longer (think "nano" seconds!) for the left ventricle to fill with blood. This would ultimately translate into less blood to going through your arteries—if your heart didn't compensate. Fortunately, it does. Studies have found that the *late surge* rush through the mitral valve in elderly people is stronger and meaner— which results in blood volume that is the same (if not greater) than in "youngsters."

But, as all-powerful and life sustaining as the heart is, it is still a muscle. And, like the muscles in your arms or legs, the heart too becomes weaker as you grow old.

The consequences of a weak heart? The poets might say a tragedy. A psychologist might label it low self-esteem. But, in literal, scientific terms, a weak heart means it isn't able to pump blood throughout your system as efficiently as it did in your youth. Your blood supply within its chambers might be the same, but your heart takes longer to contract between beats; the force that pumps that volume of blood through your arteries diminishes.

The arteries themselves have problems as well. Over time, the sleek, clean passageways that carry food-rich blood to every cell in your body get thicker (and, unlike a thick heart muscle, a thick artery wall spells trouble). Cholesterol, a byproduct of the foods you eat, accumulates on artery walls. Arteries can become clogged, making it more and more difficult for blood to "push" its way through. The result can be heart disease, hypertension, or stroke. *(See Chapter Thirteen.)*

All is not lost, however. Much of the wear and tear on your heart and arteries can be circumvented with a solid exercise program and a healthy diet. You've probably heard the diet and exercise mantra over and over again—that's because it works! A diet rich in fresh fruits and vegetables and low in fat will help keep cholesterol and triglyceride levels (both indicators of cardiovascular health) low. The U.S. Department of Agriculture recommends that you eat five servings or more of fruits and vegetables; the National Research Council suggests a diet that is 20% protein, 50% complex carbohydrates, and only 30% fat for maximum health.

Study after study shows that people who exercise stay fit longer. One study of sedentary middle-aged men who began a 6-month exercise regimen showed a significant increase in fitness. So it is never too late!

FAT CAT

The famous gambler Diamond Jim Brady liked to eat. His favorite breakfast, according to the records, was a gallon of orange juice, a quarter-loaf of corn bread, three eggs, steak, fried potatoes, grits, bacon, two muffins, and several servings of pancakes. Restaurateurs called him "the best 25 customers they ever had." Health professionals today would say he was definitely a gambler—with his life.

Receive helpful booklets on heart health from the:

American Heart Association
7272 Greenville Avenue
Dallas, TX 75231
(214) 373-6300
(800) 242-8721
www.americanheart.org

"Mood Music" or Hormonal Aging

For women there are no greater markers of the passing of time than menstruation and menopause, the former, the sprint towards adulthood, the latter, its maturity. In menopause the body has gone full cycle; monthly menstruation stops. Menopause is exactly as it sounds—the cessation of menses, or your period; it is due to the loss of estrogen. Perimenopause is the period of years, anywhere from four to ten years before, leading to this loss. During this time your ovaries stop producing estrogen as efficiently as when you were in your 20s. To compensate, the pituitary gland tries to stimulate the ovaries to work harder, to make eggs and ensure that ovulation takes place. This effort creates changes in other hormones necessary for fertility cycles. Progesterone levels drop; levels of luteinizing hormone (LH) and follicle-stimulating hormone (FSH) rise. This hormonal imbalance creates havoc in your system.

You might find yourself having a whole host of symptoms: irregular periods, hot flashes, night sweats, weight gain, intense

PMS and more mood swings, insomnia, heart palpitations, migraine headaches, and sexual dysfunction. In addition, many physicians think that the loss of estrogen also puts you at greater risk for heart disease and osteoporosis. (*See Chapter Six for a complete description of perimenopause, menopause, and other hormonal changes involved in aging.*)

But before you reach for the arsenic, all is not bleak for menopausal women—especially now. It's called Hormone Replacement Therapy (HRT), a prescription-only regimen that helps balance your hormones and replace the estrogen and progesterone your body has lost. HRT can reduce many menopausal symptoms, including osteoporosis, hot flashes, mood swings, sexual dysfunction, and vaginal dryness. (Studies have long shown that HRT can also reduce the risk of heart disease—but newer studies are finding that it might not be as effective in the first few years after menopause; more research is currently being done. The results are contradictory at times and the choice is not always easy. Ask your doctor if HRT is right for you.)

If you prefer a more natural approach than HRT, there are alternative products that you can use, such as plant estrogens, ginseng, tofu and other soy products, as well as progesterone cream made from sweet yams. Once again, check with your doctor and make the decision together.

As with most things in life, unfortunately, HRT has its flaws; it isn't the perfect panacea for all menopausal women. The fact is that HRT isn't for everyone. There is an increased risk of breast cancer in some women. If you or a close family member has had breast cancer, it's important that you tell your doctor before starting any HRT program. And, if possible, it's wise to see a gynecologist who specializes in menopause. She can help you weigh the pros and cons and make an informed, *educated* decision.

Since menopausal symptoms have an intimate relationship with your sexuality (and our now-absent fertility), they can create problems that you may find difficult to talk about, such as vaginal dryness and lack of desire. But these problems do not have to be your "secret." You are not alone. You do not have to say good-bye to a healthy sexual appetite along with your high-fat foods. Sexual problems can be modified with medication, exercise, and therapy. (*See Chapter Eleven for details.*)

Don't be embarrassed. Don't be afraid. See your doctor. A complete physical exam every year can make a difference between aging poorly and aging very, very well.

Some resources you might find helpful:

American College of Obstetricians and Gynecologists
Resource Center
409 12th Street, SW
P.O. Box 96920
Washington, DC 20024
(202) 638-5577
www.acog.org

National Women's Health Network
514 10th Street, NW, Suite 400
Washington, DC 20004
(202) 628-7814
(202) 347-1168 (fax)
www.womenshealthnetwork.org

Planned Parenthood Federation of America, Inc.
810 Seventh Avenue
New York, NY 10019
(212) 541-7800
(800) 669-0156
(212) 245-1845 (fax)
www.plannedparenthood.org

National Women's Health Information Center
(on-line resource only) www.4women.org

"Brainchild" or Neurological Aging

The brain: It's the epicenter of your intellect. Your personality. Your view of the world. Your emotions. Your reasoning behind what you see, feel, hear, smell, and taste. Your memory. All these parts of yourself come into play as you age, as your brain ages, as you experience things both more wisely and with more difficulty, with fearful anticipation and with more well-deserved joy.

Your body might gain weight as you grow old (remember that "middle-age spread!"), but your brain actually shrinks. After the age of 50, your brain loses 2% of its weight every year. This "weight loss" translates into fewer neurons, or nerve cells, to carry messages from the outside world through the brain—which, in turn, can mean less efficiency in processing information, in reaction time, in memory. (*See Chapters Four and Five for a complete description of how the brain works—and how it can go awry as you age.*)

There are also subtle changes in the patterns of your brain, in the fissures, ridges, and roadways of the brain. Dying neurons may cluster around protein substances in the brain creating what are called neuritic plaques; they may also form threadlike neurofibrillary tangles within their own cell bodies. Both these types of neuron clusters have been found in large numbers in people who have Alzheimer's disease.

Neurotransmitters are the chemicals in the brain that help conduct routine body function (such as temperature, breathing, and heart rate). They also enable you to react to outside stimuli, as well as transport, deliver, and ultimately store information from the outside world in your brain. Unfortunately, the amounts of these chemicals in your brain may decrease as you age. Lower levels of:

- *Dopamine*, which controls motor function, can mean difficulty in keeping your balance and possible Parkinson's disease.
- *Acetylcholine* can make your memory less sharp.
- *Norepinephrine* can also affect your memory—as well as your ability to handle stress and learn new skills.
- *Serotonin* can affect your moods.

But all is not grim. The brain is powerful and able to adjust to aging—just as the heart and other organs in your body do. Lower levels of certain neurotransmitters do not necessarily result in physical and emotional problems. In fact, studies have shown that people over 55 retain a great deal of their cognitive ability. We can think, feel, and make decisions as well as someone much younger—and possibly even better because we have years of wisdom and experience. We bring a richer, deeper understanding to issues, problems—and, yes—pleasure, too.

For more information, contact the:

American Psychiatric Association
Division of Public Affairs
1400 K Street, NW
Washington, DC 20005
(202) 682-6220
(202) 682-6255 (fax)
paffairs@psych.org (e-mail)

PLASTIC PARTS

Plastic not only makes your kitchen and your bath run smoother, it's also a term used for the way your brain adapts—beautifully. Plasticity means that your brain can learn new routes for transporting messages when certain neurons go awry. It means that your brain can become a "do-it-yourself" handyman, repairing, redirecting, and restoring ailing neurons—without your even being aware of it.

Brain Injury Association
105 North Alfred Street
Alexandria, VA 22314
(800) 444-NHIF
(703) 236-6000
http://www.biausa.org

American Stroke Association
7272 Greenville Avenue
Dallas, TX 75231
(800) 4-STROKE
www.strokeassociation.org

"Take a Deep Breath" or Aging and Your Respiratory System

Because your lungs are "kissing cousins" to your circulatory system, the health of your heart directly impacts on them. When you breathe in oxygen-rich air, it is your heart which makes sure that the oxygen gets to every cell in your body. Your heart also ensures that waste, in the form of carbon dioxide that leaves your cells and then travels back to your lungs. Every time you exhale, the carbon dioxide leaves your body.

As you age, your lungs lose some of their capacity. The muscles of your chest cage weaken; the tissues in your lungs become less

elastic, making it more difficult for your lungs to expand. At the age of 30, you can breathe in on average approximately six quarts of air with each inhalation. This figure slowly drops throughout your 40s until, by the time you are 50, you might inhale around four quarts of air. By your 70s, it is possible you'll only be able to breathe in 3 quarts. (This is one of the reasons why the symptoms of emphysema, a smoking-related disease in which your lungs cannot take in enough air, usually becomes symptomatic as we age. A very strong reason to quit smoking now!)

You can help stop the ravages of "air time" by beginning an exercise program. Studies have shown that older people who are in good physical condition have an oxygen consumption that equals—and even surpasses—younger, less active counterparts.

Some places to contact for more information include:

The American Cancer Society
1599 Clifton Road, NE
Atlanta, GA 30329-4251
(800) ACS-2345
(404) 325-2217 (fax)
http://www.cancer.org

National Heart, Lung, and Blood Institute
  Information Center
P. O. Box 30105
Bethesda, MD 20824-0105
(800) 575-WELL
(301) 251-1223 (fax)
nhlbiic@DGS.dgsys.com (e-mail)

American Lung Association
1740 Broadway
New York, NY 10019-4374
(212) 315-8700
(800) LUNG-USA
info@lungusa.org (e-mail)

"You Are What You Eat" or Aging and Your Gastrointestinal System

There's a reason why television commercials for heartburn and irregularity depict people who are, well, of a "certain age," people who remember when platform shoes and tie-dye were popular . . . the first time around. The reason? As you age, your gastroin-

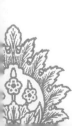

testinal tract—from your esophagus and stomach to your gallbladder and liver, from your small intestines to your colon—simply becomes more sensitive. Muscles work a little slower. Carbohydrates, protein, and fat take longer to digest. Acid production increases. In short, the wear and tear of everyday life over the years affects the efficiency of your digestive system.

The gastrointestinal tract is also susceptible to the ailments of the elderly. Heart disease can increase mucous production—which can "clog" the pathway of your food. The antacids you reach for when stomach upset, due to increased stomach acid or reflux action can compromise your immune system; they can inhibit the ability of your body to absorb certain antibiotics and heart medications. A weakened immune system, in turn, provides a perfect environment for bacteria to grow—in particular, *Helicobacter pylori* —which scientists now believe is the mastermind behind mid-life ulcers. (*See Chapter Fifteen for more information on gastrointestinal problems that can occur as you age.*)

Then there are reasons for gastrointestinal conditions that might never have occurred to you:

- *False teeth* can make you swallow more air with each breath—creating uncomfortable excess gas.
- *Gallstones*, composed of cholesterol, protein, and fat, might take years to build up—and now can create nausea and a burning sensation in your stomach.
- *Laxatives and sedatives* you might take as you age can create stomach upsets.
- *Gas*, a common ailment for women over 50, is not always a result of a sluggish, diminished capacity to digest food. The production of gastric cells have actually been found to increase in the elderly—which can translate into gastritis and upset stomach.
- *Depression* can make you lose your appetite; antidepressants can create temporary nausea and cramping.

In short, it's no surprise that gastrointestinal tract upsets affect one in very five elderly Americans. Over time, the fatty foods you eat, your sedentary lifestyle, excess alcohol and sugar, will affect the shape of your stomach and intestines.

But there is something you can do—and it's very simple: Eat less fatty foods. Get off the couch. Drink and eat desserts in moderation. The fact that gastrointestinal upsets are often caused by other conditions of old age makes it even more important to live

IRREGULARITY IS NOT A FOUR-LETTER WORD

If you feel more and more constipated as you age, you're not alone. It's a very common ailment for women in their senior years. Why? Because you eat less when you are older, and your body takes longer to digest what you do eat. Peristalsis, the "relax/contract" progression of food through your intestines, slows. And medications you might take as you age to help heartburn, anxiety, and hypertension can also create irregularity.

Some more contributing factors: Due to the uncomfortable feelings of bloat and gas that can accompany eating fibrous fruits and vegetables (the very foods that help make you regular), you might avoid anything with fiber in it—especially those brussels sprouts your mother said were good for you. You also may be prey to some "lazy" habits, including a lack of exercise and not drinking enough water—both of which can exacerbate the problem.

Constipation itself can be a cause of more constipation. The more laxatives you take, the more irregular you can become.

The solution: Make a healthy lifestyle a "regular" part of your routine. Eat more fruits and vegetables. Cook them for one minute in boiling water to make them easier on your stomach. Drink lots of water. And get moving!

in a healthy way. Start a healthy regimen now and your gastro-intestinal tract will keep "quiet" and not "talk back."

If your digestion is off-kilter, these organizations may help:

Digestive Disease National Coalition (DDNC)
711 2nd Street, NE, Suite 200
Washington, D.C. 20002
(202) 544-7497
(202) 5460-7105 (fax)
www.ddnc.org

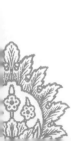

**National Digestive Diseases Information
Clearinghouse**
2 Information Way
Bethesda, MD 20892-3570
(301) 654-3810
(301) 907-8906 (fax)
www.niddk.nih.gov/health/digest/digest.htm

"Going with the Flow" or Aging and the Urinary Tract

Ah, the good old days . . . when you were able to sleep the whole night through without waking up to urinate. When you could go for hours in the car without needing a pit stop. When you could sit through a whole meeting without fidgeting because you need to relieve yourself. STOP! The urge to eliminate more frequently is normal as you get older. It is as natural and common a sign of aging as gray hair and a wrinkle or two.

Your bladder loses approximately one-half its capacity as you approach your senior years. In the same way your muscles lose their tone, their ability to "bounce back," so, too, does your bladder; it becomes less elastic. Consequently, you'll need to urinate more, pure and simple.

The urge to urinate, however, is different than incontinence—which is the actual *loss* of bladder control. Although one out of every ten people over the age of 65 suffer from urinary incontinence, *it should not be ignored.* The inability to control your bladder can be a sign of an infection; it can mean embarrassment and, ultimately, withdrawal from family and friends. You can become depressed and continually feel stressed.

The good news is that incontinence can be treated. Today medications and a wide variety of products are available to ease your embarrassment and discomfort. You can even use exercise to help control your bladder. Specific pelvic-floor "Kegel" stretches can strengthen these muscles. (*See Chapter Twelve for more information on treatments and cures of urinary incontinence.*)

The kidneys are also not immune to old age. By the time you are 70 years old, half of their filtering tubules, called nephrons, are lost. Waste is not as efficiently filtered out and eliminated through your urinary tract. To ensure healthy kidneys, make sure you see your doctor for routine examinations. Make an *immediate* appointment if you experience:

- A frequent need to urinate, accompanied by extreme thirst
- Swelling in the hands and feet
- Bad breath and a metallic taste in your mouth
- Shortness of breath, combined with extreme fatigue
- Dry, patchy, itchy skin
- A sudden loss of appetite

Any of these symptoms may signal kidney disease and, if not treated, can be life threatening.

Research has found that kidney disease in your senior years may be attributed to excess Vitamin D and protein in your diet. If you are elderly, make sure you aren't overdosing on Vitamin D with milk and too many multivitamins. And eat lean cuts of meat and fish.

Some places to contact for more information:

National Association for Continence
P.O. Box 8306
Spartanburg, SC 29305-8306
1-800-BLADDER (252-3337)
www.nafc.org

National Kidney and Urologic Diseases
Information Clearinghouse
3 Information Way
Bethesda, MD 20892-3580
(301) 654-4415
www.niddk.nih.gov

Simon Foundation for Continence
P.O. Box 835
Wilmette, IL 60091
1-800-237-4666
www.simonfoundation.org/html

The idea of your body as a temple might sound like a New Age mantra, but it's not far off the mark. Your body *is* your house, the place where your mind, your spirit, and your personality live. And, like any house, it can become and remain a comfortable and nurturing environment—as long as it is maintained, fixed when needed, restored, and kept clean and fresh. A strong, healthy body does not have to be an impossible dream. We live in an exciting time, filled with medical possibilities, scientific breakthroughs, and visionary research. You can make *your* house a home.

To that end, the next section of this book, which details the specific conditions that can occur as we age, is broken up like a home. We'll take you on a tour, inspecting each "room" of your body to see what problems can arise—and what you can do about them.

It's time to open the door and enter the house you call your body. Welcome. . . .

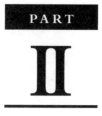

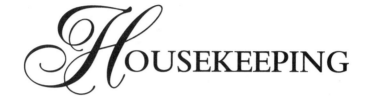

HOUSEKEEPING

4

*E*MPTY ROOMS, UNFAMILIAR VOICES: MEMORY LOSS

Second childishness and mere oblivion.
—William Shakespeare, on old age

Eileen remembered a sunny day. She didn't remember the year or the month. She didn't even remember the people she was with. But she could still feel the sun's heat on her strong back. She could see a lake, glittering in the glare of the sun. She could still hear her own laugh, her deep, rich laugh, so hard it made her shoulders shake. She remembered the warmth of a hand touching her cheek, oh so soft. She was happy, filled with joy and an absolute serenity that would never, ever die.

But that was a long time ago, far away and distant. Eileen is older now, in her seventies. She was diagnosed with Alzheimer's disease three years ago, and it has gotten progressively worse. At first, she could cover up her memory loss with a laugh or a non-committal shrug. She would ask for more detailed directions; she would leave notes for herself on every table in her apartment.

Unfortunately, Eileen got sick with a bad bout of pneumonia. She had to spend two weeks in the hospital and, during that time, her confusion, her panic, her memory loss grew worse. She didn't remember when her daughter came to visit; she saw her dead husband at her bedside, kissing her forehead.

When Eileen recovered from her illness, she was a different person. She couldn't live alone anymore; she was totally dependent. She had to move into a nursing home, where each day was brand new, like just budding trees. But sometimes, in the middle of the afternoon or in the early morning, there were glimmers of what once was.

That young laughing girl was gone. The day. The sun. The glittering lake. But Eileen could still feel, for those short few moments, the impression of that day. It was as much a part of her as her hands, the nose on her face. It was as ingrained as humming or drumming her fingers to a soundless tune. Every so often, sitting in her wooden chair in her plain room at the nursing home, Eileen could remember that once upon a time she had been young.

Memory loss is always difficult. It is a thief, robbing us of our past, the significance of our lives, entering without permission and stealing away in the night. Whether caused, as in Eileen's case, by Alzheimer's disease, or by stroke, depression, or simply the wear and tear of aging, memory loss is traumatic—for both its victims and their families who have to watch it unfold.

*M*EMORY MYTHS

Yes, memory loss is a function of aging, but it is not inevitable. Not everyone has as dramatic a loss as Eileen. The average person actually loses less memory than you might think. In fact, one particular study found that, at the age of 27, most people could recall a 7-digit phone number. No surprise here but this same study found that most people 40 years older, at the age of 65, could still recall 6 digits of that same number.

Another study, this one published in *Developmental Psychology*, used a list of 12 unrelated words to determine how much the ability to recall decreases with age. Surprise! The study showed that adults over the age of 40 recalled more words than those in their 20s—*and a large number of people in their 60s and 70s did better than the average 20-year-old.*

More good news: Vocabulary skills and general knowledge actually increase as you age—proving that experience is indeed a good teacher.

Some memory, however, will decline with age. It's a fact of life that certain cognitive abilities worsen as you grow old. Some of these include:

- *Learning new skills.* Did you ever wonder why your 20-year-old niece has already mastered the computer, but you haven't gotten beyond "power on/off?" You can blame this one on age.
- *Following directions in a strange town.* As you grow older, it takes longer to process information. You might hear the gas station attendant tell you to go right and left, but following what he told you is a whole different thing. It has nothing to do with not knowing how to drive; it has everything to do with perception and memory.
- *Getting out of the house on time.* Taking a shower. Putting on your makeup. Getting dressed. It just takes longer to get moving when you are older. Tasks take longer. Efficiency and speed decline even if your memory feels as if it is crystal clear.

These memory losses are part of what scientists call "fluid" intellectual abilities. They fall in the categories of complex problem solving, unfamiliar material, and strange new situations. There can be a decline in your fluid memory, but many times, it goes undetected. Thanks to solid life experiences and good social skills, your cognitive functions can seem intact well into your senior years. Intellectual abilities that rely on these life experiences are rock hard.

Whether or not there is a decrease in your "fluids" as you age, the way you process information and turn it into memory remains the same.

MEMORIES ARE MADE OF THIS

Put in computerese, memory is like a computer chip, processed information that is stored in a hard drive: your brain. But your individual memories are more than just data, input and output, ad infinitum. Like a good movie that sticks in your mind along with the popcorn in your teeth, your memories are infused with thoughts, smells, and emotions. Your memories are what make

you rich, full, and uniquely yourself. Memories are the embodiment of your passage through life.

But as dramatic, as poignant, as powerful, as memories can be, they all begin in a very cut and dried manner—as a scientific process.

Road Travel: Getting the Message to the Brain

Memory begins with an action, when your nerve endings receive a stimulus from the outside world— say, a hornet's sting on your right arm. The sensation of *sting* is, at this moment, an electrical impulse moving with light speed intensity. It travels up your arm, along your spinal cord, and up to your brain through a complex route of nerve cells. At the base of the brain, the electrical impulse known as *sting* stops moving merrily on its way along the great "nervous system highway." Why? It has reached a synapse, a space between the end of one neuron, or nerve cell, and another. Here, at this roadblock, the brain shows true genius. The same electrical charge that carried "the sting" now triggers the release of a chemical: a neurotransmitter. This chemical impulse is able to move across the space to receptors on the next neuron—where it turns back to an electrical impulse. The entire transformation occurs between every neuron—and it all happens at lightning speed. (*See Figure 4–1*).

The brain interprets sensations like the sting, sending out a painful "ouch!" loud and clear to travel back to that right arm. It might add a touch of fear and the need to run. The brain will also dip into its memory banks and add the newly ingrained message: hornet stings hurt.

A Memory is Born: Encoding a Message

When that first sting registers the first jolt of pain, it becomes a memory. The message that has worked its way up to the brain, crisscrossing countless other messages, bouncing back and forth from synapse to synapse, finds itself a permanent home in the temporal and frontal areas of your brain.

Acquiring information and turning it into memory is called encoding. Like a data bank on your computer, your brain files the message: "sting." And, like an efficient search engine, your brain creates links to other associations: your memory of stinging insects, your feelings about pain, that summer day when you were six and were bitten by a hornet at the picnic.

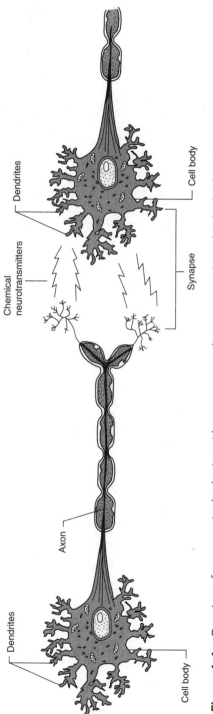
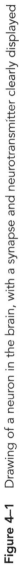

Figure 4–1 Drawing of a neuron in the brain, with a synapse and neurotransmitter clearly displayed

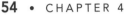

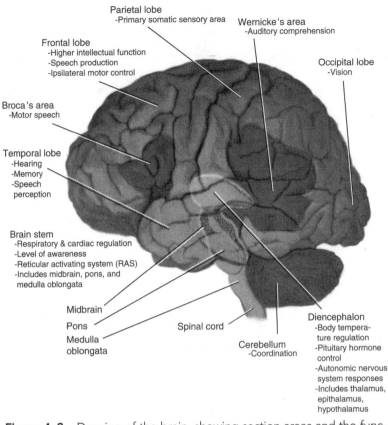

Parietal lobe
-Primary somatic sensory area

Wernicke's area
-Auditory comprehension

Frontal lobe
-Higher intellectual function
-Speech production
-Ipsilateral motor control

Occipital lobe
-Vision

Broca's area
-Motor speech

Temporal lobe
-Hearing
-Memory
-Speech
perception

Brain stem
-Respiratory & cardiac regulation
-Level of awareness
-Reticular activating system (RAS)
-Includes midbrain, pons, and
medulla oblongata

Midbrain

Pons

Medulla
oblongata

Spinal cord

Cerebellum
-Coordination

Diencephalon
-Body tempera-
ture regulation
-Pituitary hormone
control
-Autonomic nervous
system responses
-Includes thalamus,
epithalamus,
hypothalamus

Figure 4–2   Drawing of the brain, showing section areas and the functions they mastermind

These links help make memory stick. They flesh out your response and are activated the next time you are faced with another bee in the future. They create knowledge that lasts. In fact, studies show that memory loss in seniors can very well be a result of an inability to register, or encode, information when it comes into the brain.

Home Entertainment Units: Information Storage

In the same way that video cassettes keep our favorite movies and moments alive, parts of the brain keep our memories alive—preserved and ready to be added to your stimulus/reaction mix. When your brain receives a message, neurotransmitters send it to a small area in the brain called the hippocampus—the "Holder of

DANKESCHÖN—A LOT

Despite the fact that it is considered the benchmark for social security benefits, retirement, and movie house discounts, turning 65 does not automatically make you "old." Indeed, the "65 rule" is not even an American invention. In 1865, Otto von Bismarck, then chancellor of Germany, established the first social security system, using 65 as the age for benefits to begin. Considering the fact that most Germans at that time didn't live past 45, this was less an act of generosity than it was a political coup.

the Remote in the Brain Household." The hippocampus, with a chemical click, turns on the television—and memory storage banks, in the temporal lobes and other areas of the brain, become activated. Like a video cassette in the play mode, storage banks are "played," sifted through, checked, fast and furious, to find pertinent references.

Suddenly, you remember that sting at the picnic as if it had happened yesterday—not 50 years ago. You remember the fruit juice you were sipping and how it got all over your clothes. You remember crying and crying and reaching out for your mother. These perfectly preserved memories help you react to today's sting. You want to run away. You want to cry. You might even feel sticky even though you haven't had any juice. You've become that 6-year-old child again. . . .

It is problems in information storage that cause forgetfulness in many older adults. If the message their brain had received was stored more than a few hours ago, many seniors will forget it—even if their encoding abilities are intact. But all is not doom and gloom: if asked to remember something after just a few minutes, adults of every age have the same level of recall.

Picking Up the Pieces: Retrieving a Memory

Most memory problems come in the process of retrieval. Even if our memory banks are completely intact, fresh and strong, with solid information dating back to our earliest years, without

efficient retrieval, the information will lie there "collecting dust." Your computer may have a dozen things it can do, from giving you access to the web to helping you design a brochure, but, without you knowing how to use them, they might as well not be there; they are just taking up space.

Retrieval is activated by the hippocampus (that "Holder of the Remote in the Brain Household"), but it needs the right chemicals to "click and play" the right memory tapes. Neurotransmitters can bring messages to the hippocampus, but they can't continue on their way to the appropriate memory storage bank without direction. You might feel the sting, feel the "ouch!," but you won't be able to relate it back to the hornet—or to make the connection between the hornet, the bite, and the need to move your picnic to another site without the activation of your memory banks.

Further, the deeper the need to think, to delve into those memory banks, the harder it can be to activate the right "videos." Multiple-choice tests are easier to do than traditional essay questions, for example, because you have the answers right there in front of you, in black and white. The information is already accessible. But in an essay, you have to go back, back, to those memory banks, to information you had already learned and stored away. You have to make connections between memories; you have to use logic.

In other words, in many older adults, encoding is intact. Messages can easily make it to the brain. Storage, too, can be working efficiently. Memories are preserved in their appropriate memory banks. But, often, retrieval can be rusty. The memories are there, but they cannot come "alive."

Learning new information, remembering new facts, and acting in new ways also becomes harder to do because you can't retrieve your base of knowledge and experience to help understand and master them.

Now for the good news! Memory loss in older adults usually comes out as absent mindedness, forgetting where you put your keys, forgetting the name of someone you'd met a few minutes ago. *And these "senior moments" happen to everyone—even people in their 20s.* Further, experience often has more value than youthful memory. Knowing and retaining a warehouse full of facts cannot take the place of solid performance, based on mature wisdom and years of good judgment.

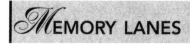EMORY LANES

Although remembering and forgetfulness both have to do with memory, there are many avenues your brain can take to get to them both:

Memory Lane #1: Sensory Store Memory

Think a blink of an eye, a few nanoseconds, of time, that's all it takes to glean sensory information and store it. These are the basic, primal stimuli, the goosebumps, the tickle in the throat, the itch that needs to be scratched, that starts our basic, primal memory going—and gets us to respond: shiver, cough, and scratch. These are the things we "remember" to do without thinking. Basically, sensory store memory is taken in without effort, simply by paying attention. It is the memory of instinct. It also functions as a waiting station, holding information until it can be acknowledged, processed, and stored in our more complex memory banks.

Memory Lane #2: Short-Term Memory

You're being introduced to a couple at a party—and now you are introducing them to someone else; you're about to take a pop quiz in an adult ed class on what you learned that day; you're telling a good friend about the movie you saw last night. These are all examples of short-term or primary memory, the information at the surface, the facts you just learned. This is the memory that hasn't yet sunk in. The all-important hippocampus doesn't get involved in short-term memory; your memory storage banks aren't activated. Short-term memory is the memory that frequently diminishes as you age. People with Alzheimer's disease lose the ability to turn this short-term memory into long-term memory. They receive information but it does not become part of their memory bank. They forget names as soon as they hear them; they forget the day of the week as soon as they are told it.

Memory Lane #3: Long-Term Memory

It takes longer for this form of memory to exist—eight seconds! That's how much uninterrupted attention is needed for the hippocampus to activate its "remote" and encode a message into its memory banks. It might not sound long, but, in reality, eight seconds is a long time for a message to take root. Long-term is what comes into play when you write a letter to an old friend or recall a dinner party from the year before. It's the memory that orders vanilla ice cream and decaf coffee, that turns down red meat and tries to lose weight by cutting out the fat. It's also the memory that can evoke past pain, past celebrations, that remembers love. This memory stays fairly intact through your life.

Memory Lane #4: Tertiary or Remote Memory

Close your eyes and picture that picnic when you were six. Think about the sky, the trees, your family's laughter, your favorite toy. Think about the hornet that dared rain on your parade. This is tertiary memory at work. Memories from long, long ago, dim with time, but, in a quick flash of windblown branches, your granddaughter's arms, the heat of the sun, come alive once more within you. Tertiary memory is always there, deep within your memory banks, needing only a specific stimulus to reawaken.

Memory Lane #5: Prospective Memory

Memories are not just conjured up from thin air. You don't just wave a magic wand and, voila!, a memory pops up in your head. It takes intellectual thought, the brain's ability to connect pieces of information, conceptualize, make deductions, and choose a mode of action. It also takes an infusion of emotion, a sprinkling of feeling, to add texture and character to a thought and a subsequent action. Combined with the brain's collection of memory pieces, a remembered emotion, an ability to move a certain way, a link to the past, you solve problems, learn a new language, figure out a way to get back to Paris.

Prospective memory deals with the future. It's memory that helps you make correct decisions and smart moves. It's the memory of experience. Put another way, it's the memory that has you remember how to call the airline to book a reservation—and how to get the best flights. It's the memory that helps you figure out the best way to save money for the trip. It's also the memory that gets you to the most convenient supermarket to buy milk on the way home from work, the one that orders pizza the way you like it from the best place in town.

Memory Lane #6: Source Memory

Memory is multi-dimensional, a rich fabric of thoughts, feelings, and facts, all linked and stored neatly in various parts of your brain. It includes not only the facts you've learned, the multiplication tables, the Internet, your favorite desserts, but when you learned them—and how. Multiplying two times two is automatic, but if you pause for a moment, you'll also remember your second-grade teacher, your textbooks, pencils, the way you stood up and spoke when it was your turn to give the answer.

Memory Lane #7: Preserved Memory

Let's go back to those multiplication tables: two times two; eight times three. The answers seemingly pop in your head, without a thought: four; twenty-four. These figures might not take a lot of brain power, but they do tap those memory banks. They are part of the information you've used over and over again, the facts you memorized so long ago. What else is considered preserved memory? Driving a car. The words to "Happy Birthday." Brushing your teeth. These tasks have been so strongly imprinted in your mind that they seem instinct more than memory. They are the "automatic pilot" of the memory chain.

Memory Lane #8: Reality Monitoring

How do you know if a certain memory is real or false? In reality, we don't always know—and can never know. Memory, like beauty, is in the eye of the beholder. Your memory of your childhood years might be different than your brother's. Your idea of how a meeting went might be very different than that of the colleague who sat on your left. But some things are part of a collective consciousness. Both you and your brother remember who your parents are, the way they read to you at night, certain television shows, meals, and trips to the store. Both you and your colleague remember the people who were at the meeting, the issues that were addressed, the clothes people wore. These reality checks help distinguish real memory from imaginary events. They are the memories that help keep you sane and grounded on Planet Earth.

These "eight lanes" on your memory superhighway combine to create a past, a present, and a plan for the future that is yours

and yours alone. These facets of memory connect and inter-twine—and sometimes collide. But they are all a part of you, as much a vital material of your "house" as your personality and the color of your eyes.

As we age, it is inevitable that we will lose some of our fine-tuning. Just as the rooms in your home might get musty, the bed-rooms of grown-up children become dens or storage bins, and your wood floors lose some of their luster, neurons die a natural death. These losses affect the all-important hippocampus. Hormonal changes, too, can affect memory.

Sometimes this is all for the good. If you remembered every single thing you learned, the details of every event, the names, addresses, and phone numbers of people you encountered throughout your life, your brain would be sorely taxed. (Talk about a headache!)

There are also times when your brain "chooses" to forget. A traumatic accident. A death in the family. Forgetting these events, at least for a while, can be a blessing.

But when memory loss inhibits your ability to remember someone you just met—or someone you love—it can be extremely painful. Forgetting dates you made just a few days ago, directions to the office that you'd called "home" for 20 years, how to fry an egg—these signs of memory loss are cries in the night.

DISTANT MEMORIES

In ancient times, age-related dementia simply did not exist. People did not live long enough to become senile. Forty-five was considered old, and people felt themselves lucky if they lived to the ripe old age of 35.

Life expectancy did not improve much throughout the years. Indeed, it took the medical and technological advances at the start of the first millennium to increase the length of our lives.

And with that longevity came all sorts of age-related diseases, from vision loss to cancer, from memory loss to dementia. But memory loss was not always as it seemed; it was not a condition in and of itself. Bacterial infections, high fever, strokes, and advanced syphilis all brought on symptoms of memory loss—which had nothing to do with age.

This holds true even today. Although we now have treatments, cures, and preventive care for many conditions, there are still subtle but direct causes of memory loss which only look like old age. These include:

- *Prescription Drugs.* Certain medications can have a "forgetfulness factor." Antidepressants such as Elavil®, tranquilizers such as Valium®, and blood pressure medicines such as Clonidine® may have a sedative effect, especially in the first few weeks of treatment. This sleepiness can affect your memory.

- *Depression.* One of the major symptoms of depression is memory loss. When you are sad, it is difficult to focus, to concentrate on the business at hand. You might ruminate, running thoughts over and over in your head—losing track of plans, names, and situations. (*See Chapter Five for the details on age-related depression.*)

- *Stress.* Remember the cliché about the absent-minded professor? Although she might very well be preoccupied with logarithms and philosophical tenets, her absent-mindedness might also be a product of too many deadlines, an upcoming faculty meeting, or college politics. Stress breeds its own brand of memory loss. Think about it: If you're anxious and nervous, how can you possibly remember the name of someone you've just met? (*Successful strategies for coping with stress can be found in Chapter Five, "Bright Walls, Solid Floors: Keeping Depression at Bay."*)

- *Physical ailments.* Hearing loss can be mistaken as memory loss. Unclear words, fuzzy-sounding speech, phrases left unsaid—these and more are often the real culprits behind forgetfulness. The same goes for vision loss: the inability to see people when introduced can make it appear as if you've forgotten you'd just met them. Chronic aches and pains can sometimes be so debilitating that you have difficulty concentrating—which can also create memory loss-like behavior. To ensure that any memory-loss symptoms you have are not actually caused by hearing or vision loss or some other physical disability, see your doctor on a regular basis. And write the dates down in your appointment book so you don't forget!

- *Hormonal imbalance.* As you read through the pages of this book, you will find that menopause can create a whole host of symptoms—including memory loss. Estrogen plays a role in normal memory function; there is a decrease in estrogen

JOIN THE CLUB

If you've walked into a room to get something, only to forget what that something is or why you'd even walked into the room in the first place, you're not alone. Sixty-two percent of all Americans have had that experience at least once in their lives. More reassuring news: A poll taken by the University of Texas found that the majority of people only remember 20% of what they hear.

production in post-menopausal women. A study of 288 women done by the National Institute on Aging found that estrogen replacement therapy can slow the decline in age-related memory loss—both visual and verbal. (*See Chapter Six for information on menopause, as well as the pros and cons of hormone replacement therapy.*)

Unfortunately, there are circumstances when memory loss is exactly that: the inability to remember, to link facts with thoughts and emotions, the present with the past. Alzheimer's disease, the ultimate memory drain, can appear terrifying—especially for those who must watch it grow in loved ones.

But knowledge can soothe the savage fear. Knowing what Alzheimer's is—and the resources available to you—can go far in providing help, and hope.

THE GREAT VOID

Dementia and Alzheimer's disease. These might be synonymous when you think of the loss of memory, but, in reality, they have separate roots. Dementia is the umbrella term, derived from the Latin words for *mind* and *away*. A physician will use "dementia" to describe mental impairment in general.

Dementia can also be caused by hardening of the arteries or multiple infarctions—a progression of mini-strokes that can occur

WHAT'S IN A NAME?

In 1906, Dr. Alois Alzheimer, a German neurologist, performed an autopsy on an elderly woman who had suffered from dementia. He noticed that many of the cells involved in memory and cognitive reasoning were bundled together like knots in a rope; he dubbed them neurofibrillary tangles. He also noticed clumps of material around these tangles; these he called senile plaques. After performing autopsies on several other demented patients who had the same brain patterns, he realized that these knot-like tangles and plaque build-up were directly related to the dementia. The medical world rewarded his findings by naming his discovery after him: Alzheimer's disease.

as you age. This is called multi-infarction dementia, which is made worse by poorly controlled blood pressure.

Alzheimer's disease (AD) is, by far, the "evil king." It is the most common cause of dementia in older people. One out of every 10 people will have Alzheimer's by the time she reaches the age of 65. That number increases to 1 out every 2 people—an alarming 50%!—by the age of 85. But there is good news: if you make it to 90, the odds are that you'll never get AD.

It certainly doesn't make people feel better to learn that the disease can be inherited. Scientists have found the gene called apolipoprotein E (APOE) is more prevalent in people with Alzheimer's disease (AD). This gene has three offsprings: E2 (which is associated with later-onset AD), E3, and E4 (which is associated with earlier-onset AD). One of the cutting-edge treatments being researched today involves giving a person with APOE-4 an APOE-2 "cocktail" which may delay the symptoms of Alzheimer's.

Another gene protein recently discovered to influence AD is bleomycin hydrolase (BH), which has been found in people with late-onset Alzheimer's. As there are no hard and fast cures yet available, being tested for APOE and BH can be an exercise in

LATE BREAKING NEWS

For years scientists have been looking at the genes that may trigger Alzheimer's disease (AD). Although promising as predictors, pinpointing these AD genes does nothing to prevent the disease from spreading. But now, as this book goes to press, recent studies have brought new hope to preventing Alzheimer's. The latest research details two enzymes—beta-secretase protease and gamma-secretase protease—that trigger the genes into deadly action. These two enzymes literally cut the Alzheimer gene's threads (amyloid precursor protein) into fragments that ultimately become the toxic AD. By studying these enzymes, scientists could very well develop drugs that block the enzymes from their "dirty work"—and stop AD before it even starts!

futility at this time. Having this gene pool does not make Alzheimer's a reality. *These genes merely make you vulnerable.*

Other factors that put you at risk for AD include:

* *Family history.* You can't escape your family at holidays—or when it comes to AD. If you live well into your 80s and have a mother, father, or sibling who had AD, you have two to four times greater the risk than the general population.
* *Your aging brain.* Normal aging reduces some of your brain power—the neurons, neurotransmitters, and synapses that make your mind work efficiently. AD reduces the amount of the specific neurotransmitters GABA, norepinephrine, and acetylcholine (ACh) even farther. In the case of ACh, the drop of 50–90% is staggering.
* *Age itself.* The incidence of AD doubles every year after a person reaches the age of 60. That figure increases by 1% between the ages of 60 and 64—and skyrockets to more than 40% after 85. (But remember: after the age of 90, your risk of AD decreases significantly.)
* *Gender.* Women live longer than men—which could explain the higher prevalence of AD among them (the "age factor").

THE WORRIED WELL

Forgetting an important date . . . losing your keys . . . becoming irritable and scattered. Like nuclear war or polluted water, the fear of Alzheimer's disease is always present, but dim. In most people, it's something that gives them a slight pang of worry every so often—nothing more. But as we age, Alzheimer's looms larger. Stress, menopause, and depression can all create "Alzheimer-like" symptoms and we can become more fearful. Unfortunately, for some, this fear becomes overwhelming. Rather than viewing life as full of possibilities, they see it fraught with fear. These people are called the "worried well." If this sounds like you or someone you know, have a complete physical to rule out any underlying problems—then seek out the help of a mental health professional. It's not impossible to turn your "worried well" into a positive "wishing well."

But studies have found that, on balance, women have a greater risk for developing AD over the age of 65. Why? In one word: Estrogen. As we have seen, this hormone has been found to contribute to good memory skills. In menopause, as estrogen levels drop, the risk for AD may climb. The good news is that hormone replacement therapy (HRT), which increases estrogen levels, may possibly slow down—and possibly prevent—the ravages of AD. In fact, the landmark Baltimore Longitudinal Study on Aging, which has observed aging in 2,000 people over 40 years, found that HRT actually reduced the risk of developing Alzheimer's in post-menopausal women by 50%. *(See Chapter Six for more information.)*

- *Head size.* There are times when a "swelled head" can be good for you. Studies have found that people with smaller head sizes are at an increased risk for developing AD. Since people with large heads have more nerve cells to begin with, they can afford to lose some—without showing signs of Alzheimer's. Like a car that has a bigger gas tank, some people have more cognitive reserve; they can go more miles with that one tank of gas than other cars.

- *Intelligence.* IQ factors also add fuel to your cognitive reserve. If you start out with a higher IQ and good cognitive skills, you simply have more "fuel" and it will take longer for the tank to show up "empty." Research supports this theory. Several studies have shown that people who have developed dementia started life at a lower intelligence level.

Although there are not yet cures for AD, there are some new medications and treatments available that can help stave off its debilitating effects, some damage control for your "home."

ℛEPAIRING THE ROOF AND CLEANING THE ATTIC

A clean home is an organized one. If your attic is uncluttered and free of dust, you'll have less of those pesky dust mites to make you sneeze, less trouble locating that old tax return, less of a mess when you want to find old pictures for your grandchildren. In the same way, your brain can benefit from less clutter, too. Here are some "household cleaners" that can help your brain remain sharp, quick, and focused—and your memory razor-sharp.

- *Prescription drugs.* There are currently four medications on the market specifically used for AD: tacrine (Cognex®), a drug with many side effects, donepezil (Aricept®), a better tolerated medication, and, the newer ones, rivastigmine (Exelon®), and galantamine (Reminyl®), which may give even better results. These drugs help increase the amount of acetylcholine (ACh) in the brain—which should help slow memory loss. Although most studies have found only little to modest improvement with these medications, every patient deserves a chance to try them. It's very possible that you or your loved one could be in that small percentage which benefits. There is no doubt that better therapies are on the horizon.
- *Estrogen.* Your doctor should give you a blood test to see if your estrogen levels have dropped. As we have seen earlier in this chapter, low amounts of this hormone can create memory loss symptoms. Conversely, the estrogen in hormone

AN HERB WITH PROMISE

Gingko biloba is not the name of your nephew's pet lizard. Nor is it an island in the South Seas. Rather, gingko biloba is a member of the fledging world of medicinal herbs. Gingko is the number-one herb prescribed in Germany for symptoms of memory loss. A study in the *Journal of the American Medical Association* found that taking 40 mg of gingko biloba extract three times a day improved cognition and socialization in patients with AD. After six months of the gingko biloba regimen, many of these same patients showed less deterioration than their non-gingko counterparts. Gingko acts as an anti-inflammatory and may expand blood flow in your brain. Can it really help? The verdict is still out. Recent reports of increased bleeding are very worrisome. Ask your doctor whether gingko biloba is safe for you—and to make sure there are no contraindications with other medications you currently take. And do not take it for at least two weeks before any surgical procedure. Gingko is a prime example of a so-called "safe and natural" supplement that can have fatal results when taken by the wrong person.

replacement therapy can give your memory a boost—up to 50% over the long-term.

- *Vitamin therapy.* It's no longer considered quackery to take a vitamin and mineral supplement every day. Vitamin E has been found to help your heart; a study from the Columbia University College of Physicians and Surgeons also found that Alzheimer's symptoms were reduced in 341 patients who were given 200 units of Vitamin E in combination with a Parkinson's drug, selegiline hydrochloride. Another fact: Vitamin B12 deficiency has been found to create memory loss in the elderly. When your mother said, "Eat your vegetables!" she wasn't wrong. All kinds of vegetables, from spinach to lettuce, are a good source of B complex vitamins.

- *Anti-inflammatory medications.* In the same way that joints and tendons become inflamed in arthritis, so do brain cells as AD progresses. Studies have shown that the over-the-counter non-steroidal anti-inflammatory drugs (NSAIDs) you take for aches and pains, such as Advil®, may actually help slow AD down as well.

- *Memory exercises.* If you are one of the millions of Baby Boomers moving towards "old age," chances are you won't be heading out to pasture like a sheep. You'll want to do everything you can to stay strong and active. That's where brain stimulation comes in. Studies have been done on aging populations which show that those who have stayed mentally stimulated throughout their lives have a lower incidence of memory complaints. In other words, take courses. Do crossword puzzles. Travel to new places. Read a book. And, if your memory has slipped somewhat, do not despair. Compensate by writing lists, keeping a routine schedule, and writing names and places down in a notebook. Consider seeing an occupational or cognitive therapist. These therapists can help you literally retrain your memory, teaching electrical impulses (read: messages) to bypass damaged neurons and use other, recently dormant pathways in the brain instead. This can help improve your everyday life.

Some places you can go to for additional information and help include the:

Alzheimer's Association
919 North Michigan Avenue, Suite 1100
Chicago, IL 60611–1676
(312) 335–8700
(800) 272–3900
www.alz.org

Alzheimer's Disease Education and Referral Center (ADEAR)
P. O. Box 8250
Silver Spring, MD 20907–8250
(800) 438–4380
www.alzheimers.org

National Institute of Neurological Disorders and Stroke (NINDS)
Public Inquiries
Building 31, Room 8A-16
Bethesda, MD 20892
(301) 496-5751
www.ninds.nih.gov

Society for Neuroscience
11 Dupont Circle, NW, Suite 500
Washington, DC 20036
(202) 462-6688
www.sfn.org

National Foundation for Brain Research
1250 24th Street, NW Suite 300
Washington, DC 20037
(202) 293-5453
www.brainnet.org

When you repair your roof, the rain won't leak inside. If you clean your attic, you'll have a clearer picture of what you store and what you can just as soon get rid of. You'll be able to retain a more organized, cleaner home. The brain, too, needs maintenance. You need to keep it active and strong. Like your home, if you take care of your brain and its mental capacities, you'll live a more comfortable, joyous life.

But what if you feel hopeless and helpless? What if you don't want to be healthy? What if your brain feels as if it is on overload? We'll be tackling depression, what we consider the walls and floors of your home, in the next chapter.

5

$\mathscr{B}$RIGHT WALLS, SOLID FLOORS: KEEPING DEPRESSION AT BAY

Happiness is no laughing matter.
—Richard Whately

Janice was not an introspective woman by nature. Give her a crisp Sunday afternoon, a tennis match on TV, some Ben and Jerry's Rocky Road, and her family gathered round, and she was a happy woman. It didn't take much.

But lately, things had gotten off-kilter. Worse than off-kilter. It began about six months ago, when Janice's husband gave her a surprise party for her 60th birthday. She remembered the feeling she had as she walked into the living room and heard the shouts of "Surprise!".

Here was shock, of course, and delight, too, at the glow on her friends' faces. But here was something else, something that filled her with terror: She would not live forever. She was going to die some day.

Janice never thought about it before, not really. She knew enough to try to take care of herself. She and her husband had joined a health club. She'd quit smoking more years ago than she could remember. And she tried not to have the steaks she loved more than once every two weeks. She did all these things out of habit, out of common sense. Prevention was important to live a good quality of life. Death itself was just an abstraction. At least for her and those she held dear.

But now it hit her like a dull weight. She was going to die sooner than later.

From that moment on, thoughts of death and dying never left her consciousness. She went to her office at the bank with death in the air. She walked her dog, the big chocolate lab she loved, worrying about dying. She ate her dinner hoping she wouldn't have a heart attack at the table. She went to sleep praying she'd wake up.

In short, Janice was in trouble. All those thoughts of dying had an impact. She felt hopeless about her life. She felt helpless in the face of her reality of mortality. She spiraled down into a depression.

Instead of enjoying her golden years, she was allowing them to tarnish. She stopped eating. She spent her nights tossing and turning in bed. She communicated with her family in monotones, with her colleagues at work by shrugging her shoulders.

When Janice lost interest in her beloved tennis matches, her husband put his foot down. "That's it. You have to see a therapist, he said emphatically. "After all, what was the point of all our hard work, raising the kids, putting money away for the future, if we can't enjoy them!"

Janice agreed. He was right. She recognized that she had changed, that she needed help. Her doctor gave her Zoloft®, an antidepressant; she also offered strategies for coping with getting older. She encouraged Janice to talk about her anxieties and fears.

Slowly, Janice began to accept the limitations of aging—and how she could work around them. She knew her memory and ability to focus was not as good as 20 years ago. The solution? Lists. All over the house. After she'd turned 60, Janice became fatigued in the afternoon. The solution? A simple nap!

Janice learned how to pare down her obligations, to make time for the people she enjoyed seeing—and make excuses to those she did not. She learned to delegate more at work. She found more time to see her two grown children—and her grandchildren.

Best of all, she once again cherished her evenings at home. With her family, her ice cream, and a tennis match going full blast.

Depression doesn't have to be a given, a fact of growing older. Yes, there is always something to be anxious about, something to worry about and fear, but it doesn't have to rule your life. Like Janice, you can recognize the signs of trouble—and do something about it. You can restore your "home" to its bright, shining past.

WHEN THE GOLDEN YEARS ARE LESS THAN BRIGHT

Whether a child, a teen, or an aging adult, the feelings of depression can be cruel. It doesn't matter if they're the result of your stolen bike, your stolen boyfriend, or your stolen youth: depression can hit anyone at any time.

Externals are only part of it, of course. There are also biochemical reasons for depression, pathways in the brain that go awry. And physical pain can create feelings of despair as potent to an 8-year-old as an 80-year-old.

But there are some triggers—"depression darts"—that are specific to seniors.

Depression Dart #1: Senior Stress

Empty nest syndrome, retirement, mortality. These are buzzwords for a generation of baby boomers. They are facts of life, experiences that almost everyone who lives long enough will face.

That doesn't make these life transitions any easier—and when you are going through them, they can hinder your health.

Some facts:

- Researchers at Georgia State University and the University of North Carolina interviewed 737 men and women between the ages of 58 and 64. Those who were still working had the highest self-esteem, while retirees exhibited more depression.
- Menopause is more than hormones. It is a physical signal that a woman is no longer young. Children who have grown up and moved away also symbolize the passing years. These life

events almost always create some sadness; so common is this reaction that it has become a cliché.

- The Centers for Disease Control have found that depression is often a precursor to high blood pressure.
- People who are depressed are four times more likely to suffer from a heart attack than those who are on an even keel.
- Women who are depressed are more at risk for osteoporosis. One study, from the National Institutes of Mental Health, found that depressed women had 11% less bone density than their happier counterparts.
- The main cause of depression in the elderly is the stress of physical illness and loss.

These sobering statistics can be enough to create stress-related depression, let alone exemplify it, but there is good news. Even though stressful life situations might be different in the elderly, they aren't necessarily harder to handle—nor do they have to take you on a downward spiral.

In fact, studies have shown that aging adults handle stress better than their younger counterparts. A study, for example, that examined both young newlyweds and aging adults between the ages of 50 and 60 found that the supposedly "carefree" newlyweds experienced more emotional distress than the seniors. In another study, this one of 375 people aged 45 to 70, found that 80% were still working, 75% had had no major illness, 94% were still married and had not been widowed, and 85% had not experienced the "empty nest syndrome." Aging definitely has its rewards!

Despite these silver linings, many older people experience emotional upheaval in their golden years; the stress they feel is difficult to handle. If this is you or someone you love, try these antidotes for stress-related depression:

- *Pro-active behavior.* The means accepting what you have to — your age, your growing children, your slower reflexes—and learning new ways to handle stress. Instead of "learned helplessness," think "learned optimism." Live in spite of losses not because of them.
- *Rather than feeling sorry for yourself, imagine yourself with all this wonderful free time*—to read, to pursue hobbies you hadn't had a chance to discover, to volunteer in your community, to enjoy.

THE THREE FACES OF STRESS

Stress doesn't always show up as anxiety or depression. It can also trigger many other emotions, as well as create very real physiological symptoms. Stress can also make you develop a whole mindset of negative cognitive thinking. Here's some examples of what stress can do—to both your mind and body. For example, physical palpitations may translate into the negative mindset, "I can't do it." It can make you feel a great deal of fear—all at the same time.

PHYSIOLOGICAL	COGNITIVE	EMOTIONAL
Palpitations	"I can't do it"	Fear
Irregular heart Rhythms (Tachycardia)	"Everyone's looking"	Panic
Butterflies in stomach	"Get me out of here!"	Fear, worry
Hyperventilation	"I'm going to die"	Panic
Weakness in joints	"I'm trapped"	Lonely, depressed
Tremors	"I should do . . ."	Angry, fear
Dizzy	"It's not fair"	Angry, sad
Dry mouth	"I shouldn't do . . ."	Depressed, guilt
Fatigue	"It would be terrible if . . ."	Shame, anxiety
Sweating	"I hate myself"	Guilt, shame
Headaches	"I'm trapped"	Guilt, worry
Insomnia	"I can't do it"	Rejected, fear, depressed, anxious
Abdominal pain	"What if . . ."	Worry

- *Stay active.* Exercise is good for the soul. A half-hour around the block can lift that weighty feeling. You may not be able to hit a 250-yard drive anymore, but you can still play golf.
- *Get a pet.* It might not be a substitute for the kids gone off to school, but think of it this way: Buttercup won't talk back. And she'll give you undying love. She needs you! Many older people have found that a dog or cat can ease their loneliness.
- *Start lifting weights.* Believe it or not, resistance training helps more than stiff bones and flaccid muscles. A Tufts University study of men and women aged 60 to 84 who lifted weights for 10 weeks found that 82% no longer felt depressed.
- *Take in a movie* or a game of cards. Making time for friends, for socializing, is not only fun, it's a great way to chase away the blues.
- *Become more spiritual.* Religion may help make you more centered; some women find it helps them cope when life circumstances feel out of control. If it's been a long time since you've visited your place of worship, plan on going in the next few weeks. You just might find some peace and newfound strength.
- *Think positively.* It can be difficult to avoid negative thoughts and behaviors. Negativism feeds on itself. Before you know it, all will feel like doom and gloom. On the other hand, positive thoughts also feed on themselves. The more positive you are, the more optimistic you'll be—and the more things will seem to go your way. Most importantly: think realistically.

Depression Dart #2: "Masked" Depression

It's not as if sad feelings come in to town like the masked Lone Ranger crying, "Hi, ho, Silver." It's not as if they creep up on you at a masked costume ball. "Masked" depression never wears such obvious, well, masks. Most times, you won't even be aware of its disguise. A by-product of some medications, illnesses, or chronic pain, this type of depression is easily wiped out—but only if you can recognize it.

Unfortunately, if you are a "golden oldie," the risk of missing the signs of depression is high. Symptoms such as memory loss, fatigue, irritability, can all be chalked up to old age or senility, when, in fact, these symptoms are a clear red flag for depression. Some of the "costumes" that disguise symptoms of hopelessness and helplessness include:

FOLLOW THE POSITIVE ROAD

It might sound like a cliché, a theory framed in smiley faces and white clouds, but if you think happy, you will be happy. It has been proven that positive thoughts beget more positive thoughts—and thinking positive thoughts is a skill you can acquire. This learned optimism is based on some very simple truths:

- *Don't dwell on the things you cannot change.* Accept them and go on. Ruminating about them will only cause more stress—and anxiety.
- *Try to think of concrete solutions to problems you may have.* If necessary, write down what's bothering you. Then step back for a moment and pretend you are only an observer. What would you do to change things? This will help you work out solutions.

- *Medication.* Some prescription drugs for high blood pressure, menopause, allergies, asthma, and pain can cause depressive symptoms. (For example, some beta blockers can cause apathy and depression.) The first place to look when new symptoms appear is in the medicine cabinet—and at the medicines you are already taking. Always check with your physician or pharmacist before taking any new medication—and make sure your doctor knows what medications you are taking at all times.
- *Brain chemistry.* Depression is not just a reaction to life's ups and downs. True, such age-related events as widowhood or retirement are tremendously stressful, but sometimes they are merely the triggers for a depression that has been lying dormant. Millions of people suffer from depression—and are genetically predisposed to succumb to it. Clinical depression has been linked to low levels of serotonin and norepinephrine, both neurotransmitters, in the brain; they are not properly metabolized and messages at the brain's synapses become skewed. (*See Chapter Four for a complete description of how the brain works.*) Anyone with depression has abnormal brain chemistry. The depression is an expression of a chemical

imbalance that should be addressed with medication. Antidepressants, particularly selective serotonin reuptake inhibitors (SSRI), have been found to alter the imbalance, not by adding levels of serotonin in your brain, but by altering the way serotonin acts in combination with other neurotransmitters. By changing the way serotonin works (or, in scientific terms, uptakes) at your synapses, your spirits are lifted and the symptoms of depression decrease. SSRIs are approximately 70% effective in clinically depressed people. Some brand names include Prozac®, Zoloft®, and Effexor®. Other antidepressants manipulate norepinephrine, another neurotransmitter that may be imbalanced when a person is depressed. Wellbutrin® is one of these more popular medications—with the added benefit of decreasing the craving for nicotine.

- *Cognitive behavioral therapy.* Medication gets you out of depression by correcting the chemical imbalance in your brain. Cognitive behavioral therapy maintains the gains and keeps you out of depression and from making the same mistakes. This type of therapy focuses on the present; it helps you identify negative thought patterns that keep you "trapped" while, at the same time, helping you learn new concrete ways to behave that will eliminate them.

HOW DO YOU KNOW IF YOU ARE DEPRESSED?

You don't have to be a rocket scientist to know when you have "the blues." You might feel weepy, sad, or irritable. You might have trouble sleeping. But, in a normal depression—one that is a reaction to a grief, a change, or sad news—these feelings will begin to lift in a week or two. Suddenly, without your doing a thing, you'll notice that your mood is better, that you are beginning to smile again, that life doesn't look so bad.

The trouble starts with less normal sadness—which isn't as easy to recognize. You might not even realize you are depressed—until the disease has taken hold. Its onset can be insidious.

Depression becomes an illness—what is termed clinical depression—if your sadness doesn't go away within a few weeks, if you find it a struggle to go to work, or function on a day-to-day basis. The symptoms of depression include:

- Excessive crying
- Extreme fatigue and no energy
- Excessive anxiety
- Inability to focus on the task at hand; unable to concentrate
- Social withdrawal from others
- Apathy toward people and activities
- Physical pain with no apparent cause
- Insomnia—or too much sleep
- Loss of appetite—or eating too much
- Extreme irritability; low boiling point
- Lack of joy in all things
- Loss of sexual feelings
- Rumination; obsessive thoughts
- Feelings of hopelessness and helplessness
- Irrational guilt
- Death thoughts including suicide
- Lack of self-esteem

If you exhibit at least five of these symptoms, you may be clinically depressed. Seek help from your physician as soon as possible.

AND NOW THE GOOD NEWS

Despite the way it makes you feel, depression is not all gloom and doom. The fact is that there is help out there, solid, real help that can make you feel better quickly. In addition to antidepressants (which we discussed earlier in the chapter), there are other treatments available. Some suggestions:

- *Professional intervention.* Not only is one-on-one "talk" therapy crucial for antidepressants to be effective, it can also work well on its own. Psychiatrists, psychologists, and clinical social workers are all licensed to help you cope better with stress, grief, and life's daily ups and downs. Check with your family physician for someone who specializes in the treatment of older people with depression—that's us baby boomers and up.

- *Cognitive therapy.* It might not sound exciting, but short-term psychotherapy works. Using logic, exercises, and hands-on worksheets, the therapy helps decrease the irrational negative thinking that comes into play when you feel hopeless and helpless. Cognitive therapy techniques are often incorporated in other types of therapy.
- *Medical conditions.* Sometimes it is not "all in your head." Hormonal imbalances, for example, can trigger such symptoms of depression as mood swings, irritability, fatigue, and poor sleep patterns. Many women experience such "red flags" when estrogen levels drop during perimenopause and menopause. (*See Chapter Six for details.*) An underactive or overactive thyroid can also be at the root of depression. Ambiguous disorders such as fibromyalgia (aching joints and muscles with no clear cause), chronic pain (such as migraine headaches and lower backache), and chronic fatigue syndrome can be double trouble: Not only are they controversial, they also mimic depression so much so that it's difficult to tell where one stops and the other starts. Further, in many cases, there is no physical evidence that the disease is present at all. What is the best way to get to the bottom of these "masked mysteries"? Find a doctor you can talk to, who will take your complaints and observations seriously. There are medications that can help your underlying conditions—if you know where to look.
- *Support groups.* Perhaps you're having difficulty adjusting to your empty nest now that the kids are away in college. Perhaps you feel you'll never get over the loss of your spouse. Or perhaps menopausal symptoms are upsetting you. Whatever the reason, you are not alone. The emotional upheaval you feel is most likely shared by many other aging baby boomers. Even more likely, there's a group of your peers that addresses these concerns. Check your local YMCA, church, school, or community center to see if a support group is meeting in your area. It can provide friendship, practical information, understanding and, yes, much needed support. (But a support group can't take the place of a licensed therapist in treating clinical depression.)
- *Antianxiety medication.* Sometimes depression comes with excess baggage: worry, nervousness, obsessive thinking, compulsiveness, or, in a word, anxiety. If you find that your mind is going a mile a minute, that you are terrified of

leaving the house, or that your accelerated thoughts are making you immobile, you might need more than an antidepressant to see you through. Antianxiety medication can help calm the fears and worries of aging that seem to haunt your days. Brand names include Valium®, Xanax®, Ativan®, and BuSpar®. *Caution: antianxiety medications can make you drowsy. They can also be habit forming and are best used for short periods of time. People who require these medications for long periods should be closely monitored by their physicians.*

• *Lifestyle changes.* It's not sexy. It's not glamorous. But it's true. A nutritious diet and a regular exercise program can help keep your body healthy. And now there's another reason—to lift your spirits. Studies show that:

• *Exercise can work as an antidepressant*—and do a lot of other good things for your body, too. When you do even light exercise—a stroll through the park, or a walk in the mall—the chemical endorphin is released in the brain. The neurotransmitter is responsible for feeling good. The more endorphins released in your brain, the better you feel. They help stop pain and keep your mood up.

• *Exercise is also a great stress-reducer.* Working your muscles will stop you from worrying. Need more convincing? Exercise will also give you more energy—which, in turn, helps quell depression. In fact, a study in Finland of 1,600 senior citizens found that those people who did not exercise were more depressed than those who did. And exercise can help your heart and bones stay healthy, too. Isn't it worth a half hour or so out of *your* day?

• *St. John's Wort.* This natural herb is used extensively throughout Europe to treat depression. It has mild SSRI properties, like Prozac®, which means that it is classified with those drugs which raise serotonin levels in the brain. Easily accessible in health food stores and pharmacies nationwide, St. John's Wort has been found to be helpful in mild to moderate forms of depression. However, a new study by the National Institutes of Health found that the herb does not help alleviate depression. The jury is still out on its effectiveness, and you should be aware that St. John's Wort is a chemical that interacts with many medications. Check with your doctor before taking this or any other herbal remedy.

FOLLOW THE POSITIVE ROAD

As children and young adults, we've always been encouraged to solve problems. To take a long, hard look at what's bothering us and do something about it. But, as we get older, that might not be possible. We might be angry that we can't move as fast as before or that our memory is a tad fuzzy, but we can't turn back the clock—no matter how much plastic surgery we book! Instead, healthy seniors learn to cope emotionally: feeling fortunate that things aren't worse . . . looking to others for support and help . . . being thankful for what they have. The emotion-focused way of coping means acceptance—and peace.

- *A diet rich in B vitamins* can help stave off the blues, especially in the elderly. Studies have found that deficiencies in the vitamin B complex can cause symptoms of depression. (One study, for example, found that 79% of people with depression had a vitamin B6 deficiency.) Get your proper dose of "the Bs" by eating lean meats, chicken, leafy, green vegetables, whole grains, beans, fish, and fresh fruit such as strawberries, apples, and oranges.

- *Taking a selenium supplement* has been found to improve people's moods when taken in regions where the soil is deficient in this mineral.

- *Alcohol has a depressing effect* on your body. You might want that drink to keep your sadness at bay, but long-term it will only make you feel worse. Drink only in moderation.

- *Caffeine and sugar can make your mood drop—fast.* That early morning coffee jolt might give you a "rush" initially, but by mid-afternoon, the only "energy" you'll feel is a wallop of fatigue.

- *Structuring your days is an asset.* Organizing your waking and sleeping patterns will help you stay focused; you'll be able to complete tasks in a timely fashion; your self-esteem will improve. How to get a routine that makes you happy? Avoid naps, try to go to bed at the same hour every night, and keep workloads on an even keel as much as possible—not too much and not too little.

WHAT DOES AGE HAVE TO DO WITH IT?

Many famous people have defied the numbers, achieving greatness well past the age of 75. Some examples:

- Margaret Mead
- Pablo Picasso
- Arturo Toscanini
- Duke Ellington

- *Be optimistic and think positively.* This cannot be said often enough. You cannot underestimate how important a positive attitude is in avoiding depression. Try to always see the glass as half full—not as half empty.

Some organizations that can provide more information:

American Psychiatric Association
Division of Public Affairs
1400 K Street, NW
Washington, DC 20005
(202) 682-6220
(202) 682-6255 (fax)
paffairs@psych.org (e-mail)

Depression & Related Affective Disorders Association (DRADA)
Meyer 3-181
600 North Wolfe Street
Baltimore, MD 21287-7381
(410) 955-4647
(410) 614-3241
www.drada.org

National Institute of Mental Health
Information Resources and Inquiries
5600 Fissthe Lane, Room 7C-02
Alexandria, VA 22314-2971
(703) 684-7722
(800) 969-NMHA
(703) 684-5968 (fax)
www.nimh.nih.gov

We hope the chapter has given you some insight into the nature of depression—and how it can dim the walls and floors of your soul. We also hope it has given you the tools you need to get help, to learn how to make these years truly golden. *(You'll find more lifestyle "golden nuggets" throughout the book.)*

Now it's on to another "room" in your house, one that is closely linked to your moods: hormones and the endocrine system.

6

ℋORMONE INSULATION

Life should be lived as play.
—Plato

Ten years ago, Miriam went for her yearly physical, fully expecting that she'd get the same clean bill of health she'd always received. The doctor checked her heart; he checked her blood pressure. The nurse drew blood. The doctor asked Miriam if she'd had any symptoms she wanted to talk about.

Miriam shook her head. She didn't think so. She felt great. True, she was a little bit more tired than usual and she had developed a habit of carrying bottled water around with her, but that didn't seem to be a problem.

There was one thing, however, that she didn't want to share with her doctor. She felt too embarrassed. The past few months had brought some unpleasant changes. She had kept getting urinary tract infections, a condition that is often nicknamed the "honeymoon disease" because it can occur with frequent intercourse. But it wasn't as if she and her husband were newlyweds;

they'd spent 35 happy years together and, at this stage of the game, quality was more important than quantity. But even quality wasn't particularly great. The few times they were intimate had been disappointing. Miriam had felt pain; it was as if her infection had decided to stay, no matter how many antibiotics she took. Her husband said it didn't matter, but it had bothered her; she'd never had such discomfort before. To add insult to injury, Miriam felt the need to urinate almost every half hour. She felt frustrated and anxious—adding to the stress at work and the emptiness she felt now that her last son had gone off to college. Whatever it was, Miriam didn't want to discuss it with the doctor—yet. She just chalked it up to growing old, empty nest syndrome, and stress.

Over the weekend, while Miriam was waiting for the results of her blood test, she felt more tired than ever. All she wanted to do was eat and drink—and nap. Her husband was growing concerned; he wanted to take her to the emergency room. Miriam refused.

Monday morning arrived. Miriam called her doctor and found out that, along with millions of others, she had adult-onset Type 2 diabetes; her body was resistant to the insulin she produced and could not control her blood sugar level. In Miriam's case, it was less the high blood sugar itself that was a problem, but complications—heart disease, kidney failure, and blindness. In fact, Miriam had "Syndrome X"—a combination of diabetes, elevated blood cholesterol, obesity, and atherosclerosis (hardening of the arteries).

But there was light in this "sugar-clouded lining." Fortunately for Miriam, her doctor felt that the diabetes could be controlled through diet and exercise. She was told to lose weight by eating a diet that was high in complex carbohydrates and low in fat. She began a walking program, briskly moving around the perimeter of the neighborhood park three times a week.

Several months later, Miriam's condition had improved. Her weight was down, and her blood sugar was balanced. Her symptoms—the fatigue, the excessive thirst, the recurring urinary tract infections—had all but disappeared. In fact, Miriam felt better than she'd ever had in her life.

It sounded crazy, but Miriam felt that her diabetes was the best thing that ever happened to her. It had given her a second chance.

ℬETWEEN THE WALLS: ENDOCRINE EFFICIENCY

"I'm running on adrenalin in the office these days."
"My moods have gotten away with me. My hormones must be having a field day!"
"I feel so fat and tired. I bet I have a thyroid problem."
"Thanks to insulin imbalance, I now have low blood sugar."

Adrenalin. Estrogen. Thyroid production. Insulin. Hormones take on almost mystical power in our understanding of medicine. We blame their imbalance on everything from stress and depression to fatigue and weight gain. And, indeed, sometimes a hormonal problem is behind our condition—especially as we age.

Getting older not only affects your circulatory and nervous systems, your digestion and your bones, it also may create havoc in the chemical mix that makes everything work: your hormones.

Think of your hormones as your thermostat, the stuff that keeps you warm and safe, calm and cool. They are your regulators, your furnace and your cooling system, your protection against the elements. Thanks to the hormones in the endocrine system, your home can stand up to the years.

The Greek word "hormone" means "to excite"—and the hormones, or chemicals, in your body do get you excited—excited, stimulated, and charged up. Hormones literally create action; they enable you to function.

These life-sustaining chemicals are made and stored in your endocrine glands—but some of these glands are more equal than others. Your pea-shaped pituitary gland—the master gland—located in your brain, is responsible for regulating other glands to produce hormones. It demands estrogen from your ovaries at certain times of the month. It tells your pineal gland, located nearby in the brain, to release melatonin to help you sleep. It orders your thyroid gland, at your throat, to stir up your metabolism with thyroxin—and to get your adrenal glands, located near your kidneys, to release adrenalin. (By the way, don't confuse these hormone-regulating glands with your lymph glands; they have another purpose—to swell and respond to infection.)

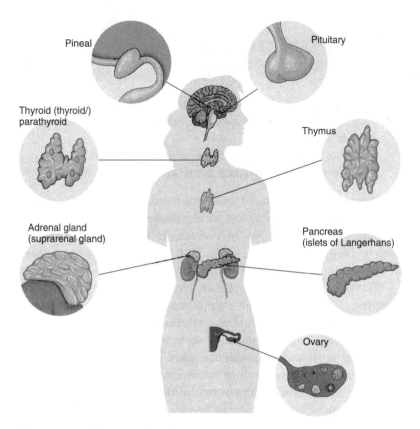

Figure 6–1 The glands of the endocrine system

Although there are many hormones that make up your home's insulation, there are four that are most critical to aging:

Hormone, Sweet Hormone #1: Growth Hormone (hGH)

This hormone says it all: growth and development. Made by the pituitary gland, hGH gives you a strong body and hard muscles; it makes you stand tall in your teens. Unfortunately, hGH output diminishes with age, especially after 40. Many scientists believe that this decrease in hGH is the reason behind aging, why growing old brings some physical and psychological deterioration; they also believe that the loss of hGH is the cause of a weakened immune system. If this is true, then an infusion of hGH should stave off the debilitating symptoms of aging. Indeed, this

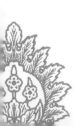

hypothesis has kept many researchers' passion "young"—and it continues to be tested in laboratories across the globe.

You can actually get injections of hGH—at a cost of approximately $15,000 a year. Although some celebrities swear by hGH infusion, long-term results have not been tallied; side effects can include high blood pressure, abnormal swelling, diabetes, and heart failure. Is hGH therapy worth the risk? Only time will tell.

Hormone, Sweet Hormone #2: Melatonin

This is another "designer" hormone, one that decreases with age and taken by people to increase their odds for longer youth. Manufactured by the pineal gland in the brain, melatonin is responsible for your regular sleep/wake patterns. Some people who travel frequently swear by it; they take melatonin to avoid jet lag.

Some researchers claim that melatonin also works as an antioxidant, protecting your body from roaming free-radical molecules that can damage your body. (*See Chapter Fifteen for more information about antioxidants and your skin.*)

Studies have recently shown that melatonin has antioxidant benefits, strengthening the immune system against disease, but they are not conclusive. In addition, taking melatonin supplements may create confusion, headaches, drowsiness, and blood-vessel constriction.

A better antiaging remedy? A healthy lifestyle, including a diet rich in fruits and vegetables and regular exercise. This will ensure that you get the antioxidants your body needs—as well as deep, dream-filled sleep.

Hormone, Sweet Hormone #3: DHEA

By itself, this hormone isn't much to write home about; it's what it "subcontracts" that is key. Dehydroepiandrosterone, or DHEA for short, is produced in the adrenal glands; it is then broken down by your body into estrogen and testosterone, the hormones associated with masculinity and femininity.

From about age 30 on, your body produces less and less DHEA—which, in turn, affects your production of estrogen and testosterone. Decreased estrogen signals menopause; decreased testosterone can affect women sexually (as well as create prostate problems in older men). (*You'll find more about menopausal conditions in the next chapter.*) Conversely, too much estrogen has been

associated with breast cancer, and too much testosterone can lead to facial hair and heart disease. Your body, at least during the developmental years, creates a balance between too much and too little. Things change as you age, and your doctor may suggest estrogen replacement therapy if you are a woman; she may also suggest medications to increase testosterone if you are experiencing sexual dysfunction.

DHEA can be purchased over the counter as a supplement. Many swear by its ability to increase energy and enhance sexual performance. The truth is that we don't know if it's safe. DHEA has the potential to create too much estrogen and testosterone in your body; the DHEA converted into estrogen can create a greater risk for both breast and uterine cancer. As always, check with your doctor before trying *any* over-the-counter supplement.

Hormone Sweet Hormone #4: Insulin

Before the discovery of insulin, people lived only two or three years after being diagnosed with diabetes. It is a miracle hormone when produced in the body—and, as a supplement, it can help women with diabetes live long and productive lives.

Insulin is produced naturally in the pancreas and then stored in the liver. When you eat, the gastrointestinal tract begins to break food down into smaller particles as soon as you open your mouth and start to chew. Starting with the saliva and taste buds in your tongue and traveling past your stomach acids, the foods you eat become smaller and smaller particles until, in the intestines, they are broken down into the smallest molecules of food your body's cells can digest. This form of food is glucose (or sugar)—and it needs insulin to let your cells know it's "dinnertime."

Insulin is like a lock and key. Insulin is the key that opens the door to muscles and allows glucose to be taken in and used. Think of it as a "dinner bell."

As you age, the dinner bell can get rusty. Your body doesn't realize it's time to eat. Basically, your pancreas can slow down its production of insulin or actually get out of synch and release the insulin too late after food is taken in, when it won't do any good. (You can also be born with a genetic predisposition to lose the total ability to secrete insulin which results in childhood, or Type 1, diabetes. Often called childhood diabetes, this label is a misnomer since it also occurs in adults.)

Your body can also become insulin-resistant as you get older. In this case, although insulin is in your bloodstream waiting to go into action, for some reason the receptors on your cell don't "see" it; they don't recognize the blood sugar and it isn't taken into the cells. Consequently, blood sugar levels rise in your body—which can lead to Type 2 diabetes.

Insulin resistance (and its resulting diabetes) is a very common condition in people past 40. In fact, if you have an insulin imbalance, you are in good company. Almost 16 million Americans have diabetes. A large number do not even know they have the problem. Don't be one of them. (*Read more about this condition later in this chapter.*)

These hormones might make your "home, sweet home," but it isn't the end of the world when, as you age, they become imbalanced. In fact, imbalance is sometimes the natural order of things. . . .

ⲆIABETES DOESN'T HAVE TO BE DISASTROUS

Remember Miriam, the woman at the beginning of this chapter who was tired, thirsty, and touchy and didn't know why? We learned that she had adult-onset (or Type 2) diabetes—and that she had to change her life.

Diabetes isn't a signal of erosion; it doesn't mean that you have to check into an old-age home. Rather, it is a condition that must be watched and treated. As simple as that—which is good news for the millions of people over 50 who are diagnosed with adult-onset diabetes every year.

When you become diabetic, it basically means that your cells have become insulin resistant; the hormone cannot do its job of converting glucose, or sugar, into energy. (*See the section on insulin later in this chapter for a full explanation of what diabetes is.*)

Unfortunately, this buildup of glucose can have dire consequences. Unchecked, excess blood sugar can damage your heart and its blood vessels; it can create havoc in your kidneys, your nervous system, and your eyes. In fact, diabetes is the number one cause of noninfectious adult blindness in this country and the number one cause of nontraumatic limb loss. It is also the number one cause of kidney failure in people on dialysis.

Hyperglycemia, or excess blood sugar, can lead to a condition in which your body, desperate for fuel, tries to break down fat for energy. The result, thanks to an insulin and glucose imbalance, is a toxic buildup of acid in your blood. Called ketoacidosis, this condition can be life threatening. More common is a "hyperosmolar state" that can develop gradually and lead to severe dehydration and confusion.

If you have been diagnosed with diabetes, hyperglycemia, or any other insulin-related condition and develop any of these symptoms, call your doctor immediately:

- Severe nausea
- Extreme weakness and fatigue
- Body chills
- Abdominal cramps
- Rapid breathing

Diabetes is tested with a simple blood test taken after a single 12-hour (at least) fast. If your blood sugar is greater than 125 mg, chances are you have diabetes. If your blood tests show up positive for diabetes, do not despair. There are many treatments available that allow you to control your condition—and not the other way around.

Dealing with Diabetes #1: Lifestyle changes

One of the most effective ways to control diabetes is in your hands—literally. Get them busy putting on your sneakers for a brisk daily walk. Exercise helps control diabetes.

And after your walk, continue to keep those hands busy by cutting up vegetables and fruit and slicing multi-grain breads. In fact, a high-carbohydrate, high-fiber diet will help cut insulin demands of diabetes by 75% to 100%. In other words, piling on the complex carbs will release glucose into the bloodstream more slowly than other foods.

But note the emphasis on complex carbohydrates. This doesn't mean cake and pizza and mashed potatoes. Because diabetes has been linked to obesity, you may need to lose weight—and that means concentrating on starches, such as high-fiber cereals and breads, without the fat.

The way you eat—and when—will also help you keep the right balance between insulin and glucose in your blood. The best plan? Three small meals and three or four snacks a day.

Sweets, as you might suspect, are *verboten*. They will not only stop you from losing weight, but they will also make your blood-sugar levels soar. Sugar can also exacerbate circulatory problems—as will smoking. High proteins continue to be controversial so be sure to check with your doctor first.

For many, learning to add an aerobic type of exercise for thirty minutes, 3–4 times a week, is the most difficult. Since exercise is critical to effective management of diabetes, try exercising only ten minutes at a time. New studies show this is just as effective as an hour in the gym.

Changing to a healthier lifestyle—one that includes a low-fat diet and smoke-clear lungs—will have immediate positive results not only on your insulin levels, but also your moods, your energy, and your overall sense of well-being.

Dealing with Diabetes #2: Medication

Some people will need only to start a diet and exercise program to control their diabetes. But others might not be as fortunate. The good news is that there are exciting, new medicines out there that can work successfully; new medicines are being developed all the time. One group increases the body's sensitivity to its own insulin; these include Glucophage®, Actos®, and Avandia®. (Glucophage® also decreases the sugar produced by your liver.) Another group works by stimulating your body to release insulin (Prandin®), while still another decreases the breakdown of sugars in your intestine (Precose®, Glyset®). Some diabetics will need a different type of medicine; they might need the help of pills that stimulate your body's release of insulin, such as glipizide, chlorpropamide, or glyburide. (If you find these names "hard to swallow", not to worry. Your pharmacist will know them—and the brand names are "easier on the tongue.") Some women who have Type 2 diabetes will need actual insulin to control their blood sugars, while all patients with Type 1 require insulin injections.

Dealing with Diabetes #3:
Don't Forget to Brush Your Teeth

Because of the blood-sugar imbalance in your body, diabetes can affect your gums and teeth. Be sure to brush twice a day—and floss. You don't want to lose your winning smile!

DINING THE DIABETES WAY

If you've been diagnosed with diabetes, don't despair. You can easily control your condition with some easy "food rules" that don't feel like deprivation:

1. **Opt for low-fat cheese** instead of the high-fat variety (which hinders your cells' ability to use insulin efficiently).
2. **Think high fiber:** whole grains, cereals, breads, beans, and muffins. A study of over 65,000 women found that those who ate the most fiber had the lowest incidence of diabetes.
3. **Get fishy over salmon and sardines.** High-fat catches of the day have been found to help prevent diabetes by making cells more efficient in gobbling up glucose.
4. **Munch on fresh fruits and vegetables.** The more apples, oranges, celery, carrots, squash, and other tasty garden treats you eat, the more fiber—and the less fat—you'll get into your system. You'll also be stacking up antioxidants that are healthy for your heart and immune system.
5. **Keep away from sugary, high-fat desserts.** A piece of chocolate cake might sound delicious, but it will raise havoc with your blood sugar—and create insulin imbalance. If you just can't seem to stay away from that dessert, try this compromise. Take a bite, not a whole serving. Limit yourself to special occasions only. It gets easier. The less sugar you eat, the less you crave it.
6. **Watch your salt intake** if your blood pressure is too high.

Dealing with Diabetes #4: Feet Smart

It might sound condescending, like telling you to tie your shoes, but being careful with your feet is crucial if you have diabetes. Nerve damage can make the smallest cut or bruise deadly. You might not feel a cut and it can become infected. Diabetes also creates circulatory problems in your feet—which can make any infection or cut difficult to heal. To avoid the spread of infection, examine the bottoms of your feet daily. Look out for red spots, blisters, cracked, dry skin, and swelling. Trim your toenails straight across to avoid ingrown toenails. And wear comfortable, supportive shoes—especially when you walk!

Dealing with Diabetes #5: Pressure Cooker

Controlling your blood pressure is one of the most important ways to handle your diabetes. Along with blood sugar management, blood pressure that is controlled is critical for organ preservation in diabetics.

For more information about diabetes, write or call:

The American Diabetes Association
1660 Duke Street
Alexandria, VA 22314
(800) 232-3472
www.diabetes.org

American Association of Clinical Endocrinology
www.aace.com

YOUR THYROID: A LITTLE GLAND WITH A BIG MEANING

The thyroid gland, nestled just below your Adam's apple, looks like a little butterfly unfurling its wings. Innocuous looking, yes, but it packs a wallop, regulating your body's metabolism and producing hormones that influence every organ and every cell in your body. When your thyroid gets out of whack, your body is sure to follow.

Unfortunately for women, they are five to eight times more likely to get thyroid disease than men—and it is a condition that

occurs more frequently as people age. In fact, by the age of 60, 17% of women may have an underactive thyroid (or hypothyroid) condition—which can increase the risk of heart disease and raise cholesterol levels.

Some of the symptoms of an underactive thyroid include:

- Mood swings and depression
- Weight gain
- Dry, flaky skin and hair
- Enlarged thyroid
- Fatigue
- Difficulty concentrating
- Trouble swallowing
- Cold intolerance
- Hoarse voice
- Bloating and constipation

An overactive thyroid (hyperthyroid) condition can also increase the risk of heart disease, as well as lead to osteoporosis.

Some of the symptoms of an overactive thyroid include:

- Irritability and nervousness
- Tremors and muscle weakness
- Weight loss
- Insomnia
- Enlarged thyroid
- Vision problems
- Depression

It can be difficult to diagnose a thyroid problem because it is often masked as something else: depression or simply the signs of menopause itself. If you suspect a thyroid problem, see your doctor, especially if you are approaching menopause. A doctor can perform a simple series of blood tests called thyroid function tests (T3, T4, TSH or Thyroid Stimulating Hormone) to determine whether your thyroid is producing within normal ranges. If your thyroid level is low, a daily pill may solve the problem. High thyroid levels may require destruction of the thyroid gland by radioactive iodine or by surgical removal.

One important note: If your TSH level test is above normal, but your other thyroid tests are at the low end of normal, you may be experiencing a subclinical thyroid problem—common in the aging population—which may require medication. Caused by Hashimoto's thyroiditis, an inflammatory disease of the gland, a subclinical thyroid condition creates a situation in which you exhibit symptoms of hypothyroidism, even though your tests show you are within normal ranges. You might have trouble losing weight. You might feel listless and tired. Your skin might be dry and flaky. If your symptoms persist, have your doctor reevaulate your condition; you may need help. (Since subclinical hypothyroidism progresses to actual hypothyroid disease within four years in approximately 20 to 40% of people, you certainly don't want to neglect it!)

We hope this chapter has helped you learn how to control your hormones—and keep your home's insulation humming. But women get a larger dose of hormonal change as they age. Menopause, as well as other specifically female conditions, deserves its own "wing." Let's go to the "new construction" that occurs in a woman's midlife cycle.

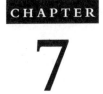

NEW CONSTRUCTION: MENOPAUSE, MAMMOGRAMS, AND MORE

When one door of happiness closes, another opens,
but often we look so long at the closed door that we do not see
the one that has been opened for us.
—Helen Keller

Life had been getting very difficult for Marlene. It wasn't the situations in her life that caused her stress. No. It was the way she had almost out of the blue begun to handle them. First of all, there were the commercials. Suddenly, she found herself weeping at Kodak™ moments; she began to reach for the tissues whenever a puppy or a child appeared on TV.

But it didn't stop there. Marlene found herself crying as she wheeled her cart down the supermarket aisles. She cried when one of her friends left for a short vacation. And she cried whenever her husband or children said seemingly innocuous remarks. "Can't we have dinner now, Mom" or "Honey, can you change the station on the radio?" sent her in a tailspin.

Unfortunately, the problem wasn't just her crying. It was her yelling. Marlene would get upset and angry at the slightest thing: a half-full laundry hamper, an unimportant message that had mistakenly not been given to her at work, a crinkled magazine. Forget about it! Marlene's tears would turn to rage and she would yell at anyone within range.

Marlene's husband, of course, got the brunt of her irrationality. He was more than upset; he was angry and frustrated. He wondered if Marlene and he should go to couples therapy; he wondered if their marriage was in trouble. But he was afraid of Marlene's reaction if he brought it up.

Marlene wasn't exactly thrilled with her mood swings, either. She hated that she couldn't control herself or her moods. She wondered, in turn, if she was crazy, if she was "cracking up." Because Marlene was in her early 50s, she thought perhaps she was in menopause; she'd read enough about the subject to know the symptoms. In addition, menopause was no longer that "dark secret rite" women had to go through alone; she had had numerous conversations with her friends about it. But it couldn't be menopausal: Marlene still got her periods—even if they were less frequent.

Instead, things went from bad to worse. Marlene's moods were soon accompanied by night sweats; she woke up drenched several mornings a week. Finally, a symptom Marlene could recognize. Perhaps she really *was* in menopause.

Marlene made an appointment with her gynecologist. The first thing she did was order a blood test to see if Marlene was still producing estrogen. The results came back a few days later: There were still levels of estrogen in her body.

Marlene started to panic. Maybe she was crazy after all. But her gynecologist assured her that lower amounts of estrogen in the body can produce menopausal-like symptoms. Marlene was actually in perimenopause.

It wasn't in her head. Marlene's lowered estrogen levels created her mood swings, her night sweats, and her irregular periods. The gynecologist gave Marlene low-dose birth control pills to decrease her symptoms.

Marlene laughed at the pink vinyl package. She hadn't seen these in a long while—and she doubted she could get pregnant at this point. She really didn't see the need for birth control pills.

But the gynecologist reassured her. These pills were not designed for birth control; indeed, they don't offer enough protection. Rather, they give your body a low dose of estrogen every day—enough to stop Marlene's symptoms in their tracks.

It was like a miracle. Almost from the first day, Marlene felt better, more in control of herself. She was calmer, happier—and she didn't wake up sweaty in the middle of the night. Her periods became regular again and she felt great. The family went back to normal.

Marlene knew that she couldn't take the birth control pills forever. Her gynecologist wanted her to stay with them for a year; they would test her FSH levels again at that time. But for now, they did the trick. Marlene was her old self again: hopeful, happy, and confident.

Marlene is not alone. Millions of women every year go through exactly the same mood swings, night sweats, and irregular periods that she suffered. The good news is that there is something women can do about it.

Aging doesn't just affect your estrogen levels, however. As you age, you also become more at risk for breast cancer; you can get cysts in your breasts, ovaries, or cervix. In the same way you watch for every wrinkle in your face, you need to be up on your gynecological exams and mammograms. Taking care of yourself is not just a luxury: it can be crucial to your good health.

In this chapter, we will go over some of the conditions specific to women, the signs and symptoms of our house that can't be overlooked with a "slap of paint," but, rather, need a fresh, new wing.

MENOPAUSE: A NATURAL— AND NORMAL—SIGN OF AGING

Twenty years ago, the word *menopause* was never uttered in polite conversation. As late as ten years ago, women suffered in silence. But today menopause is out of the closet. With millions of baby boomers turning 50 this year alone, menopause has not only found a voice—it's being shouted in every magazine, book, and television show.

Menopause is a natural function of a woman's body. It should feel no more shameful than the onset of menstruation. It's even better: With menopause, women can make informed decisions; they can be educated. Who can say the same about that first period back in grade school!

Literally, menopause means the cessation of menses (the menstrual cycle). In actuality, menopause is not what creates the usual symptoms: the irregular periods, the hot flashes, the sweats, the mood swings. Rather, it is the decline in estrogen in the *years before menopause,* (perimenopause), that can make you feel as if you've lost control. Once you're officially in menopause, the symptoms have usually diminished or stopped.

As menopause approaches, your ovaries slow down their normal functions, including the production of eggs and the production of estrogen and progesterone, the hormones that regulate monthly cycles, fertilization, and pregnancy. The decline in estrogen is usually what gives menopause its bad name; it is responsible for hot flashes, mood swings, night sweats, irregular bleeding—as well as more serious conditions, such as osteoporosis and heart disease.

The most common symptoms of menopause include:

- **Hot flashes,** starting from the head down. Seventy percent of women get them, and they can last anywhere from 30 seconds to 15 minutes at a time.
- **Night sweats,** which usually last from three to five years.
- **Irregular bleeding.** Not a reason for concern unless the bleeding is heavy, or a period lasts more than 7 days, or menstruation cycles are less than 21 days apart. Irregular bleeding can be a sign of fibroids, polyps, or something more serious. See your doctor!
- **Insomnia.** Sometimes the inability to sleep through the night, a function of aging, creates the irritability and mood swings some women experience.
- **Weight gain.** A fact of life as you get older, especially if you are sedentary. The best solution? Exercise and eat right.
- **Migraine headaches.** If your migraines begin during menopause, hormone replacement therapy (HRT) may help ease the pain. But if you've had migraine headaches for your whole adult life, HRT might make them worse—and also add other symptoms, such as nausea and bloating. Check with

your doctor if your headaches stop you from enjoying your day-to-day activities.

- **Heart palpitations.** Rapid heartbeat often accompanies a hot flash. If you've had anxiety attacks before menopause, it's possible they'll get worse. But antianxiety medication and estrogen can alleviate the fear.
- **Loss of concentration.** Memory loss can be a sign of aging (*see Chapter Four*), but it can also be a result of other conditions such as insomnia, anxiety, or depression. Since menopause can cause all of these conditions, which came first? The chicken or the egg? The memory loss—or the sleeplessness from menopause? We might not have the answers, but we do know that estrogen helps keep you focused.

Hormone replacement therapy (HRT) can take away many of your menopausal symptoms. In the 1960s, when hormone replacement therapy was first introduced, doctors prescribed estrogen alone. It was found, however, that when taken alone estrogen can increase the risk of uterine cancer by 20%. It may also increase the risk of breast cancer. Today, HRT consists of a pill or patch that combines estrogen and progestin (a synthetic form of the sexual hormone progesterone). Although progesterone can cause some PMS-like symptoms, its addition to HRT is well worth it. Progesterone reduces the risk of uterine cancer so much that it becomes insignificant. It offsets the risk of breast cancer as well.

What can you expect with HRT? A great deal. Menopausal symptoms, such as mood swings, insomnia, hot flashes, headaches, aching joints, and an inability to concentrate, can all be improved within two weeks of starting HRT. In addition, HRT helps your skin's elasticity, making it less dry and wrinkled as you age.

But the most important benefit of HRT may be its ability to prevent osteoporosis and heart disease. (Studies are also finding that HRT may also reduce the risk of colon cancer.) In fact, some studies have shown that HRT can decrease heart problems by almost 50%. Another study, at the University of California at San Francisco, has shown that women with only modest levels of estrogen will have two and a half times less hip or spine fractures. Still other studies have found that estrogen therapy can slow down Alzheimer's disease and macular degeneration in the eye.

While these studies are encouraging, other studies question the benefit of HRT in heart disease. One study has found that heart attack risk is raised the first two years of HRT. The ongoing Women's Health Initiative has found that even heart-healthy women can have a heart attack or a stroke within the first two years of HRT; since this study is ongoing, future findings may ultimately find that HRT is heart healthy from day one. Because the final answer is not in yet, check with your doctor to determine what is right for you.

MENOPAUSE MYTHS

Myth #1: Forget about sex after menopause.

Fact: On the contrary, many women find menopause liberating. Think of it: No more messy periods. No more birth control. It's true that vaginal dryness can be a result of estrogen decline, but there are many over-the-counter preparations that can take care of the problem quickly and quietly. If you are experiencing a lack of desire, it can be caused more by life stress, such as the "empty nest" and aging parents, than by menopause.

Myth #2: Women get crazy during menopause.

Fact: True, some women have a more difficult time of it than others—just as some women experience severe PMS while others go through their cycle without a problem. Depression itself is not a result of menopause, but serotonin levels, responsible for many mood disorders, can become imbalanced during the time of hormonal change. The best solution is plenty of exercise and a healthy diet—and, if symptoms are severe, ask your doctor about an antidepressant or hormone replacement therapy.

Myth #3: Menopause is always a hard time.

Fact: Wrong! In reality, only 25% of women have symptoms that need additional interventions. Even more interesting: in countries where age is a respected, venerable part of life, women experience much fewer symptoms.

As with any medication, HRT takes some getting used to. Some women report feeling bloated and crampy from the added progestin; they might also get monthly vaginal bleeding. Other women feel nauseous from the estrogen. Your doctor can adjust the dosages to help prevent these side-effects. There are also several different types of HRT. You can either take an estrogen pill every day and a progestin pill for only 12 days a month, or a combination pill in which you take both estrogen and progestin every day in what is called a "combined-continuous" therapy. This combination pill has had much success in stopping vaginal bleeding.

THE OTHER SIDE OF THE HRT CONTROVERSY

So if HRT is so great, why doesn't everyone take it? As with anything in life, there are cons along with the pros. In this case, the major con is a higher chance of breast cancer. In fact, if you have a strong or immediate family history of breast cancer, HRT is not recommended.

Further, even adjusting the dosages of HRT might not alleviate your symptoms—or your uncomfortable side-effects. In these circumstances, you may want to investigate natural ways to reduce menopausal symptoms.

Some natural ways to manage menopausal symptoms:

* **Phytoestrogen, or plant estrogens,** can be found in things that grow; biochemically, they are identical to synthetic hormones but produce fewer side-effects.
* Some of the **natural supplements** that might help heart palpitations, vaginal dryness, and hot flashes include:

    Black cohosh (especially good for hot flashes)
    Wild yam cream (which might help mood swings)
    Chaste tree ointment
    Vitamin E supplements (Studies have also found this may be an effective weapon against heart disease.)
    Calcium supplements (All women should take 1,500 mg. daily.)
    Garlic (Tablets won't have the odor you encounter when cooking—and they may help lower cholesterol and blood pressure in menopausal women.)

- **Soy products,** such as tofu, are an almost perfect food for women in menopause. They contain phytoestrogens (those healthy plant estrogens) that studies have found can help reduce hot flashes as well as your risk of osteoporosis, high cholesterol, and breast cancer. Other soy foods include soy milk, soy nuts, and soy beans. Aim for one or two servings, or one cup, daily. One word of caution: try to get your soy from foods. Soy supplements contain very high concentrations of phytoestrogens and may raise your risk of breast cancer.
- **Exercise** will help alleviate your menopausal risk of osteoporosis and heart disease. Try to get your heart pumping for at least 10 minutes several times a week, via walking, a treadmill, bicycle riding, or a home-gym stairstepper. Lift three- to five-pound weights at your gym or at home for strength-training exercise. Strong muscles will increase your flexibility and help prevent bone loss.

Natural remedies and lifestyle choices or HRT? Or a combination of both? The choice is yours. Make it an informed one by finding out as much as you can about menopause. Talk to your doctor. Here are some useful numbers and addresses to help you during your menopause information quest:

American College of Obstetricians and Gynecologists
Resource Center
409 12th Street, SW
Washington, DC 20024
(202) 638-5577
www.acog.org

Human Development Resource Council, Inc.
3941 Holcomb Bridge Road, Suite 300
Norcross, GA 30092
(770) 447-1598
(770) 447-0759 (fax)
www.hdrc.org

*K*EEPING ABREAST

Breasts, along with the reproductive organs, change as you age. Shape is one factor; as you age you lose elasticity in your breast tissue. Another factor, and one that is not as visible to the eye, is the increased risk of breast cancer after menopause.

In case you were wondering if there was any good news about menopause, the decrease in estrogen means that breast pain can often go away—as well as cysts and lumps that may have plagued you starting in puberty.

When you menstruate, estrogen levels increase. This brings more fluid into your body, including your breasts. Just as your belly might feel bloated, so too can your breasts. This swelling expands and stretches the nerves in your breast—and can make them feel tender and painful. The decrease in progesterone at this time can also cause pain.

The low-dosage birth control pills or HRT you might be using during menopause can also contribute to breast pain. The influx of estrogen creates the same fluid retention and swelling as it did when you used to get your periods.

Cysts or lumps can also make your breasts feel painful. Ironically, the tumors associated with breast cancer usually are silent and deadly. You don't feel any pain at all.

The medical term for lumpy or cystic breasts is fibroadenosis, or fibrocystic disorder; they are connected to the hormonal changes in the menstrual cycle. What does this mean as you age? The same as it does for breast pain: cysts disappear as your estrogen does.

It goes without saying: if you feel any lump in your breast after menopause, call your doctor immediately and have it checked.

BREAST CANCER FACTS

Breast cancer is the most feared form of cancer for women—even though new studies show that women are at a much higher risk for heart disease than breast cancer.

But the numbers are still sobering:

- One out of eight American women develops breast cancer.
- It is the most common cause of cancer in American women.
- Over 180,000 new cases are discovered every year.

Do not despair. To offset these shattering numbers, there are excellent positive ones:

- Breast cancer today has a high cure rate: 97% of all women survive at least five years after early detection.
- The death rate for breast cancer has steadily dropped over the past 5 years for Caucasian and Hispanic women.

- More and more women recognize the need to speak to their doctor if they discover a lump. They no longer "hide and deny." This early detection can save their lives.

Ironically, breast cancer is most prevalent in postmenopausal women—whose estrogen levels have decreased. Here, it's not a question of hormonal activity in the present; it's the years in the past when menstruation was a monthly occurrence, a hormonal clock.

Estrogen, a reproductive hormone, tells your cells to divide; that is what it is designed to do. But the more cells divide, the more the chances that abnormal cells will crop up. The more years that go by, the greater the chance of abnormal cells, or cancer risk.

Of course, age is only one factor. There are other critical risks that you should be aware of:

- A family history of breast cancer
- Benign breast lumps or cysts
- A previous bout of breast or ovarian cancer
- Menstruation beginning before the age of 12
- Bearing a child after the age of 30
- The onset of menopause after 55
- A menstruation cycle that is longer than 29 days or shorter than 26 days
- Taking birth control pills (This risk factor is controversial. Most studies have found that the pill has no effect at all in whether or not you get breast cancer. In fact, some women actually went into remission when they started the pill.)
- Hormone replacement therapy (Also controversial.)
- A high-fat diet
- A sedentary lifestyle

The best way to help prevent breast cancer—or catch it in the early stages—is with a mammogram. (A monthly breast self-examination and a yearly clinical breast exam by your doctor are also important.) This is a low-dose X-ray of the breast that shows the appearance of lumps up to two years before you could possibly feel them.

Many physicians suggest a baseline mammogram between the age of 35 and 40. This X-ray serves as a reference for future mammograms; a radiologist can compare X-rays and see if there has been any change, however subtle, in your breast tissue.

THE BREAST CANCER GENE

Gene research has enabled scientists to isolate the gene that may cause breast cancer among family members. A mutation in gene p53 or BRCA 1 or the presence of gene BRCA 2 have been pinpointed as the breast cancer genes. About 1 in every 200 women carry one of these. But before you seek out a genetic counselor, remember that having the gene does not mean you will absolutely get breast cancer —only the fact that you are predisposed to getting it. It is not etched in stone.

If your mother or sister or daughter did indeed have breast cancer and genetic testing shows you have the gene, then yes, the predisposition is high. In these rare cases, you might consider strong preventative measures, such as a mastectomy—but only after careful deliberation and conversation with your doctor.

Both the American Cancer Society and the National Cancer Institute recommends a mammogram every year for every woman over the age of 40. This is especially important if you are post-menopausal and on any form of hormone replacement therapy. If you are in a high-risk group, you should have a mammogram starting ten years before the age it was detected in your family member.

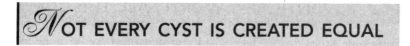

NOT EVERY CYST IS CREATED EQUAL

The lump you may feel in your breast does not automatically spell cancer—although any lump should be checked by your doctor as soon as possible. A benign cyst usually feels slippery; it's easily moved around when you touch it. A cancerous cyst, or tumor, is usually harder and thicker; it might cause some dimpling on your breast skin.

The best way to feel a lump is, well, to feel it. You should give yourself a breast self-examination every month. The best time? In the shower, after soaping up, to smooth your skin. Here's how:

1. Check your breasts for any dimpling.
2. Raise your arm and using your fingers, apply light pressure in a circular motion, moving from just at your armpit towards your nipple. You are looking for tiny surface lumps. (Use the right fingers to check the left breast, and left fingers to check the right breast.)
3. Repeat, this time using firm pressure to feel any possible deep lumps.
4. Squeeze your nipple to make sure there is no discharge.
5. Repeat the same examination on your other breast.

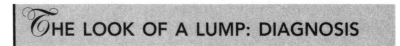

THE LOOK OF A LUMP: DIAGNOSIS

If your mammogram shows a lump, it doesn't automatically mean you have cancer. Your doctor will usually have a sonogram done; this is an image of your breast that is created with ultrasonic sound. Here your doctor can determine if the lump is filled with fluid or if it is solid—and if further testing is needed.

A needle aspiration (or core biopsy), a procedure done in your doctor's office or in the radiology suite, takes material from the lump so that it can be sent to a laboratory for diagnosis. An excisional biopsy, done only in surgical surroundings, can determine more accurately if the lump is cancerous or not.

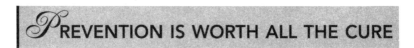

PREVENTION IS WORTH ALL THE CURE

Although genes cannot be spliced and destroyed (yet!), there are many risk factors of breast cancer that can be fixed.

You Are What You Eat

A low-fat diet, rich in fruits and vegetables and whole-grain cereals can help keep breast cancer at bay. Instead of butter, use olive oil. Think low-fat milk and other dairy products. Fish instead of saturated fat meat. Grilled foods instead of fried.

Smoke Begone!

Yes, yet another reason to put that cigarette down now. Women who smoke are also at a higher risk for breast cancer.

Exercise Your Might

Brisk exercise a few times a week can help reduce your chances of breast cancer—not to mention help your mood, improve your circulation, and keep heart disease at bay. Why not try one of those charity walks to raise money for breast cancer research?

Drink in Moderation

Studies have shown that alcohol can increase the risk of breast cancer. But other studies have shown that one glass of alcohol a day can reduce your risk of heart disease. The best solution? Stick to one glass. This way you can have your "cake" and enjoy it, too!

Think Yearly

When it comes to gynecological exams, the word leap year does not exist. Make sure you see your doctor every year for a mammogram and complete gynecological exam. The life you save may be your own.

Cutting Edge Medications

Two drugs now on the market have been found to actually reduce your risk of breast cancer. Both tamoxifen (Nolvadex®) and raloxifen (Evista®) have been found to keep estrogen levels at bay. They are used primarily after a cancer has been removed and a patient has then tested positive for estrogen receptors.

For more information on breast health, contact:

The Susan G. Komen Breast Cancer Foundation
5005 LBJ Freeway
Suite 250
Dallas, TX 75244
(972) 855-1600
(972) 855-1605 (fax)
www.komen.org

American Cancer Society
1599 Clifton Road, NE
Atlanta, GA 30329-4251
(800) ACS-2345
(404) 325-2217 (fax)
www.cancer.org

𝒯HE OTHER SEXUAL ORGAN: YOUR OVARIES AND AGING

Your ovaries work hard over your lifespan. During the menstrual cycle years, each of these almond-shaped organs contain thousands of eggs waiting to be fertilized. During each cycle, one or more of these eggs grows in a small kernel-like structure known as a follicle. In ovulation, the egg becomes mature and the follicle ruptures. The follicle turns into a minute structure called the corpus luteum; the egg is released and it floats down to the uterus via the fallopian tubes.

But that's only part of their duties. Month after month, the ovaries produce estrogen and progesterone (as the egg follicle ruptures and becomes a corpus luteum); both help thicken and prepare the uterine walls in case one of its eggs are fertilized and needs a "room."

Problems can arise when an egg follicle or a corpus luteum continues to grow rather than disintegrate after the egg is released. Fluid can build up, forming cysts (known as polycystic ovary syndrome).

𝓔VERYTHING YOU WANTED TO KNOW ABOUT FIBROIDS

Fibroids might sound like some kind of whole-grain, sci-fi asteroid, but, in reality, they are a mass of abnormal tissue. In other parts of the body, they'd be called tumors. Because they are found in the pelvic region, scientists simplified matters by calling them fibroids. They usually develop between the ages of 35 and 45; about 40% of women past 40 develop them. If you are overweight, your chances

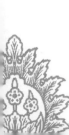

of developing a fibroid increase. And, for some reason, they are more common in African-American women.

Although they are usually confined to the uterus, fibroids may "invade" a nearby organ if they grow too large. If you have a fibroid, chances are you have more than one; they are also usually found in multiples. But, occasionally, a woman's uterus can grow a single fibroid that becomes so large—as big as a grapefruit — that it needs to be surgically removed. Fibroids can on occasion weigh as much as 25 to 90 pounds!

Why fibroids? Physicians aren't quite sure, but a common theory connects them to a woman's abnormal reaction to estrogen—although studies show that taking birth control pills, which contain high amounts of estrogen, may actually discourage their growth. HRT, however, may increase fibroid risk.

A FIBROID IS A FIBROID IS A FIBROID

When it comes to fibroids, location determines the type:

Submucous fibroids grow just beneath the uterine wall lining. They can create menstrual pain and bleeding. Eventually this type of fibroid may develop a stalk called a pedicle. The pedicle remains in the uterus, while the fibroid detaches itself and may actually float in the uterus or the vagina. This situation can cause pain, irregular bleeding and infection.

Intramural fibroids are found in the uterine wall.

Subserosal fibroids grow on the outer wall of the uterus. They are usually asymptomatic, causing no pain or discomfort—until they grow large enough to "annoy" other organs. When subserous fibroids grow stalks, they become . . .

Pedunculated fibroids, which can get twisted and cause tremendous pain.

Interligamentous fibroids grow sideways between the ligaments of the uterus. They can interfere with the blood supply trying to reach the uterus.

Parasitic fibroids attach themselves to other organs. They are the rarest type found in women.

Fibroids might sound scary, but they are almost always benign. Most women don't even know they have them. Problems may arise, however, when the presence of a fibroid interferes with your physician's ability to do a complete pelvic exam. And, because fibroids can sometimes be mistaken for ovarian tumors, especially if you are experiencing any kind of pain, your gynecologist will usually do a sonogram, using ultrasound scanning, to see exactly what's what. If she still isn't sure, she might do a hysteroscopy to actually see inside the uterus. An even more in-depth diagnostic tool is a sonohysterography; in this ultrasound procedure, the uterus is filled with sterile water to provide better scanning.

Although most women are symptom free, fibroids can sometimes cause:

- Excessive bleeding
- Pain
- Swollen abdomen (which is not really the belly—it's the uterus stretching and pushing up on the intestines)
- Infertility

More good news for menopausal women: Fibroids usually shrink and disappear after menopause. But occasionally they need to be removed surgically. Discomfort, abnormal bleeding, sudden enlargement, or the location and type of fibroid may indicate that it needs to be removed. There was a time when a hysterectomy was almost a common procedure. Fortunately, today there are other ways to ensure the safe removal of a tumor:

A *myomectomy* can remove each tumor individually without harming the uterus or the uterine wall. (This is especially important for a woman who may later want to try to get pregnant.)

A *hysterectomy* becomes an important option when the fibroids are increasingly growing larger and a woman is in menopause. It is an operation that involves the removal of the uterus. Because the ovaries remain intact, it is possible that a premenopausal woman will not experience menopause immediately after the operation, but follow her natural course.

Drug therapy can also work in reducing fibroids. Lupron® Snarel® and Zoladex® contain gonadotropin-releasing hormones which decrease the blood supply to the uterus—and starve out the fibroids. These medications are taken either as a self-injection or as a nasal spray. The only drawback is that the tumors usually grow back after you stop taking the medication. And, if you are not yet in menopause, the medications can accelerate the process and create menopausal symptoms.

To learn more about fibroids and the uterus, contact:

National Women's Health Network
514 10th Street, NW Suite 400
Washington, DC 20004
(202) 628-7814
www.womenshealthnetwork.org

We hope this chapter has helped you learn how to work with the hormonal changes that affect your sexual being as you age. We hope your "new wing" is one you can enjoy many peaceful nights and days. It's time now to move on and take the next step—literally.

CHAPTER

8

$\mathscr{S}$TEP BY STEP: MOBLILITY PROBLEMS

Be not sick too late, not well too soon.
—Benjamin Franklin

Way back when, Maggie had been a brilliant sailor. She'd handled a skiff better than the kids she hired to crew for her. But ever since she'd turned 60, her movements had slowed. It wasn't because she was frail or forgetful; it wasn't that she'd suddenly become uncertain of herself. It was because of pain.

Every time Maggie had to use her hands, whether to tie a knot, change a sail, or even open a jar of tomato sauce, she felt pain—blinding, sheer white, aching pain.

It had begun to grow worse as her 63rd birthday approached. Her hands hurt in the rain; they hurt in the cold; they hurt in the shower. Worse, she began to feel so crippled that she was afraid she couldn't hold onto the bannister at home or in her office; she was afraid of falling down the stairs.

Although Maggie had spent her whole adult life pushing back the clock, she suddenly felt old. To her body's aches and pain, she added her head. She became depressed; she talked about the "old days" when she was young and sailed her boat in races. She stopped going to her office, a law firm she'd helped found, and spent a large part of her days staring out the window.

If Maggie's husband hadn't intervened and called the doctor, she might have spiraled down so far that she'd become suicidal. Luckily, their family doctor had known them for years. She recommended Maggie get into a geriatric evaluation and management program (GEM) at the local hospital. There, a treatment team, including a geriatrician (a physician who specializes in the elderly) and a nurse evaluator trained in assessing older patients' problems and needs, as well as a host of therapists and physicians would develop the right program for Maggie. After her evaluation, the psychiatrist on the team treated Maggie's depression with antidepressants; the geriatrician treated her arthritis with the newest anti-inflammatory drugs. The nurse evaluator recommended Maggie contact the Arthritis Foundation to find support groups, information, and strategies to help her best cope with her pain.

Just shy of her 70th birthday, Maggie had a lot to cheer about. Her depression had lifted about the same time as the pain had disappeared. Sure, she got a twinge now and then, but she had learned to recognize the signs, to accept them and not make them worse than they were. She is no longer afraid of falling—although she realizes that her days of solo sailing are behind her.

But Maggie didn't have to say bon voyage to sailing completely. For her birthday, Maggie's grown son bought her a beautiful, new windbreaker for her to wear as his first mate in an upcoming race.

Maggie's story has a happy ending, but the arthritis scenario does not always have an upbeat conclusion. One out of four Americans over 50 suffer from some type of arthritic condition—that's 16 million people in all. Some of these people may become so debilitated by their condition that they grow old before their time; they may become fearful, dependent, and depressed.

The fact is that we take walking, from one room to the next, up the stairs and down, to and from the store and the parking lot, for granted—until something happens.

And it makes sense. Why shouldn't we be on automatic pilot when it comes to mobility? After all, it is as much a part of our basic core as breathing, eating, and sleeping.

When pain strikes, the automatic pilot shuts down. Suddenly we have to think about our mobility all the time—from walking to the bathroom to walking over to the television set to pick up the remote. But pain does not have to mean that you can't continue your daily life. There have been tremendous inroads made in treating arthritis, as well as other conditions that affect your ability to get around.

In this chapter, we'll take a look at some of the more common mobility problems—as well as the different treatments available to help you get the spring back in your step.

I USED TO DANCE

If you can't walk up the stairs in your own house because your legs hurt, you don't much care what arthritis really is. All you know is that you can no longer do the things you used to do, the everyday tasks that you used to take for granted.

But arthritis is much more than those aches and pains in your arms and legs—and if you can take the time to decipher it, you can learn how to better treat it. With education comes understanding. And with understanding comes strength.

Taken from the Greek word *arth*, for joint, and *itis*, for inflammation, arthritis is really a generic name for over 100 different conditions that cause stiff, painful, and sometimes swollen joints.

Although scientists can't pinpoint to one trigger, one "broken step in your home" that causes arthritis, they do know that there is a mix of ingredients, "sticks and stones," that can cause it. These include:

Sticks and Stones #1: Old Age & Osteoarthritis

Words that often sound long-winded and complicated become clear if you happen to know Latin. Osteoarthritis, for example, sounds more serious than it is—until you apply Latin. *Osteo* means bones and, quite literally, osteoarthritis is inflammation and pain in the joints of your bones.

If you are one of the 16 million Americans who suffer from osteoarthritis, you know it. You literally live it, sometimes every day, sometimes only when inflammation flares up.

Osteoarthritis is caused by years of stress on the weight-bearing joints of your hands, your hips and knees, your feet, and your

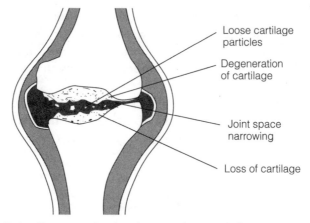

Loose cartilage particles

Degeneration of cartilage

Joint space narrowing

Loss of cartilage

Figure 8–1 Drawing of a joint bone with osteoarthritis

lower back. The stress of playing competitive sports, exercising in improper sneakers, lifting and carrying heavy bundles too many times a day—all of these and more can cause your cartilage to weaken. Add a genetic predisposition and too much weight for your body to carry, and it's possible you can develop osteoarthritis. Over time, the cartilage along the surface of your bones literally begins to deteriorate; particles of cartilage break up; bone spurs can crop up at your joints and create stiffness and pain.

Sticks and Stones #2: Your Autoimmune System, Antibodies, and Rheumatoid Arthritis

Let's go back to Latin for a moment for yet another type of arthritis, rheumatoid arthritis, and how it is connected not to your bones, but to your body's first line of defense: your autoimmune system.

In Latin (a supposedly dead language), *auto* means oneself and *immune* is part of your immune system, that vast network of antibodies and white blood cells that fight off invading viruses and bacteria. In an autoimmune disease, such as rheumatoid arthritis, your body literally battles your own cells. Here's how this self-defeating phenomenon works:

1. A virus or bacterium enters your body, perhaps from an open wound, the air, or something you ate.
2. Lymphocytes, cells similar to white blood cells that live in your lymph nodes, recognize that a foreign object (read: germ) has entered your body and sounds the alarm.

3. As much as bacteria tries to "disguise" itself, your lymphocytes can see through the masquerade. The stud-like protrusions on the surface of the "bad" cell, called antigens, do not
look the same as those protrusions on your own "good"
cells.

4. When a new virus or germ enters your bloodstream, you
might get sick; your lymphocytes don't recognize strangers.
But, once you've gotten the measles, or a cold, or that winter flu, your body won't let it happen again. New lymphocytes are made, ones that can "lock on" to the studs of that
no longer strange virus. You become immune to that particular strain of germs. (All total, your body has approximately
2 trillion lymphocytes, ready and willing to fight for you.)

5. Sometimes, however, your lymphocytes don't recognize a
cell as one of its own. The studs seem unfamiliar and your
body goes after it—as if it were an enemy. Some strep
germs, for example, look very much like heart muscle cells.
If an antibiotic doesn't kill off all the strep germs that caused
your sore throat, it's possible for your lymphocytes to "go
after" heart cells—resulting in rheumatic fever.

Although the above explanation is somewhat simplistic, this is
basically what happens in autoimmune system diseases such as
rheumatoid arthritis and lupus.

Approximately 2.5 million people have rheumatoid arthritis
(RA), which, like osteoarthritis, attacks the joints of your extremities. But, rather than causing cartilage deterioration, RA creates
inflammation in the joint tissues. It can also affect the tissues
around your heart and lungs. This inflammation causes the pain
and stiffness associated with arthritic disease.

RA can take different paths in different people. Sometimes it
can affect just one joint, your hands, say, or your ankles. Or it can
affect all your joints at once, making it difficult to walk and get
around. You also may lose weight, get a fever, feel extra tired, and
possibly get inflamed red bumps or nodules at your knuckles or
your elbows, where RA is particularly painful.

Sticks and Stones #3: Uric Acid Buildup and Gout

Contrary to popular opinion, gout is not necessarily a disease of
kings. Henry VIII, obese and self-indulgent, might have had a bad
case of gout, but it doesn't mean that you'll start killing your wives
if you have it! Nor does it mean you've lived an unhealthy life.

The facts: gout is a type of arthritis that, instead of involving your cartilage or autoimmune system, involves your metabolism—specifically, the uric acid your body produces as waste. Under normal conditions, this uric acid (which is the by-product of an amino acid called purine found in such foods as red meat, wine, beer, and sardines), dissolves in your blood and is eventually passed out in your urine. When you have gout, this uric acid doesn't dissolve; it builds up and settles into your joints. Since your lower extremities, especially your big toe, have the most acidic-concentrated joints in your body, the excess uric acid usually zeroes in on that area. Eventually, the uric acid forms crystal-like needles that send up a red flag to your immune system. Fighter cells storm your big toe and break up the crystal needles which, in turn, creates inflammation, swelling, and a great deal of pain.

Gout occurs in episodes, usually after too much "partying" or strain from walking. More men than women get it, but it affects more than 1 million people—from kings on down. Although diet is a factor in getting gout, so, too, are taking diuretics (which are prescribed for high blood pressure), obesity, and heredity. If you have gout on top of osteoarthritis, the pain from your arthritis

IF YOU'VE BEEN DIAGNOSED WITH LUPUS . . .

Although not arthritis, lupus can have arthritic symptoms. In fact, in many ways, it mirrors rheumatoid arthritis. Fever, pain, fatigue, and weight loss are all symptoms of lupus. If you've been diagnosed with this disease, which is more common in women than men, you might also get a butterfly-shaped rash on your cheeks. Lupus, like rheumatoid arthritis, is an autoimmune system disease; it inflames joints, skin, and, in more serious cases, internal organs such as the kidneys. Fortunately, many inroads have been made in this disease in the past few years. Eating right, exercising regularly, taking anti-inflammatory medicine, getting plenty of rest, and even joining a lupus support group will go far to ensure you live a happy life in your golden years!

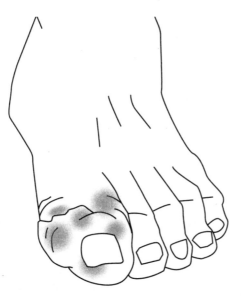

Figure 8–2   Drawing of a foot with a big toe with gout

might disguise the fact that you have gout and make it difficult to diagnose.

Sticks and Stones #4: Genes and You

Fate isn't always etched in stone. If you have a predisposition to heart disease, a healthy lifestyle will help reduce that risk. Similarly, if one of your parents or a close relative had osteoarthritis or gout, you can fight getting it by keeping your weight down, by doing strength-training exercises to make your muscles and your joints strong, by wearing comfortable shoes, and by eating a healthy low-fat diet.

But heredity does play a role—and to be forewarned is to be forearmed. In recent years, scientists have discovered that people who develop arthritic conditions have cells with a certain identifying characteristic: HLA protein. If you have this protein, it is even more imperative to maintain a healthy lifestyle.

Another factor: studies have found that estrogen has a cushioning affect on your joints. If you are postmenopausal, estrogen replacement can help ward off arthritis and gout—especially if you have a family history of joint disease.

$\mathscr{P}$UTTING THE BOUNCE BACK IN YOUR STEPS

If you are suffering from arthritis, the world might look bleak. You can't walk to the store the way you did. Your arms and legs ache. You can't find a comfortable position in a chair or even in your bed. You feel old.

Stop! There is help—solid, safe help. Here are some "stairways" to health:

Stairway to Health #1: Think Analgesics and NSAIDs

No, this isn't an encryptic language. Nor is it a solution from outer space. NSAIDS, or Non-Steroidal Anti-Inflammatory Drugs, are one of the most effective and safest ways to deal with your arthritic pain.

The most common NSAID is plain old aspirin. It can significantly reduce pain and swelling in your joints.

NSAIDS, however, have some drawbacks. They can irritate your stomach, cause internal bleeding, and, especially in people over 60, elevate your blood pressure and harm your kidneys. Even though you can purchase NSAIDs over the counter at your local pharmacy, make sure you are under a doctor's care to prevent any problems. Over-the-counter NSAIDs include ibuprofen (Advil® and Motrin®), and naproxen (Aleve®).

Acetaminophen, or Tylenol®, is an analgesic. It can be very effective in reducing pain, but it won't help your inflammation or swelling. But if you are allergic to aspirin or have an ulcer, Tylenol® can be very helpful in controlling your pain. Fortunately, the newer medications like Vioxx® and Celebrex® seem to be better tolerated and easier on the stomach. (Your doctor may have to balance these drugs with other medication that reduces stomach acid.)

NSAIDs will also help the inflammation caused by gout, but allopurinol (Lopurin® and Zyloprim®), which lowers uric acid production, is prescribed more frequently.

Stairway to Health #2: Steroid Treatment

Sometimes NSAIDs just don't do the job. Your joints are sore and swollen; your pain is intense. In cases like this, your doctor may prescribe a steroid. No, these aren't the types of steroids that

STAYING IN ONE PIECE

Falling is one of the leading reasons for disability in seniors. It is one of the most common accidents for those in their senior years. But falling is not always an accident—nor is it always your fault. As you age, you might not see as well as you once did. You might not hear warning sounds in your environment as clearly. You might not find your balance as easily; as you age, your feet become less sensitive. And, when you stand up from a chair, your blood vessels don't respond as fast as in your youth. You might feel dizzy as blood drains from your head—and lose your balance and fall. Arthritis, with its accompanying stiffness and pain, might prevent you from responding as quickly as you need to when a throw rug or an electric cord gets in your way.

In addition, your balance may be affected by the medicine you are taking—as well as by the age-related conditions you might have developed. Diabetes, heart conditions, neurological problems, even anxiety and depression might make you feel "off-kilter"; your fear of falling can make your balance problems worse. Some solutions:

- Get a thorough physical. Find the root of your balance problems. Perhaps it's a cataract, high blood pressure, or diabetes—all of which can be helped with the right medication or surgery.
- Make your house fall-proof. Get rid of throw rugs, scattered cords, icy porches, poor lighting, and store important item where you can reach them.
- Find your own pace. Be practical and use your common sense. If it's freezing cold outside, chances are you'll find ice. Go slow. Wear shoes with solid traction. And bring a cane, if necessary, for balance. Similarly, don't just jump out of a chair. Take your time.
- Start exercising. Stretches will help you become more flexible—and less inclined to fall.

exclude you from the Olympics. These steroids can effectively reduce inflammation—and any potential damage to your joints. In addition, steroids help suppress the immune system, which is particularly helpful for autoimmune system types of arthritis, such as rheumatoid arthritis and lupus.

As with any prescription medication, steroids have potential side effects. If your doctor prescribes a corticosteroid, you might experience weight gain, nervousness, increased appetite, and mood swings. Let her know immediately if you have any of these symptoms after starting your medication.

Corticosteroids can be injected directly into the painful joint or taken in pill form. The most common steroids used to treat arthritis are prednisone, cortisone, dexamethasone, hydrocortisone, methylprednisolone, and Kenacort®.

Stairway to Health#3: Try DMARDs— along with Your NSAIDs

Quick! What does DMARD stand for? If you said, "Disease-Modifying Anti-Rheumatic Drugs," congratulations! This group of medications can ease inflammation and slow down the symptoms of rheumatoid arthritis. Originally used to treat malaria, DMARDs are stronger than NSAIDs and corticosteroids, but they are slow acting. For this reason, they are usually taken in conjunction with NSAIDs.

If your joints haven't responded well to steroids or NSAIDs, DMARDs might be a good choice—as long as you don't have kidney or liver disease. Some side effects may include nausea, loss of appetite, upset stomach, diarrhea, or mouth sores. If you experience any of these symptoms, contact your doctor immediately.

Some DMARDs on the market include hydroxychloroquine (Plaquenil®), methotrexate (Rheumatrex®), sulfasalazine (Azulfidine®), and gold—yes, gold—which can be injected into a muscle (Solganal®) or taken in pill form (Ridaura®).

Stairway to Health #4: Alternative Steps: Magnets, Cartilage Pills, and Red Hot Chili Peppers

Although many of the alternative medicines available have not been scientifically proven to work, they don't necessarily harm people either. Physicians believe in the motto, "First, Do No

AND YOU THOUGHT IT WAS ALL IN YOUR HEAD

Studies have found that the same antidepressants that ease depression and anxiety can work well in reducing the pain of arthritis. In lower dosages these antidepressants have been found to block messages of "pain!" to the brain. They also help you sleep—and a good, solid rest can go far in managing your pain.

Harm." And, if the following treatments (usually harmless) provide even a modicum of relief to you, go for it!

- **Magnets.** Although there is absolutely no scientific proof that magnets will help with arthritic pain, one study has shown that they may help. Pain patients at Baylor University School of Medicine who strapped magnets on to their arthritic joints felt better after 45 minutes of "magnetic therapy." And the *American Journal of Pain Management* reported in 1999 that people with chronic foot pain who put magnetic soles in the bottom of their shoes felt better. Are magnets worth trying? Yes—as long as you don't use them as a substitute for proper medical care.
- **Glucosamine chondroitin and sulfate.** These natural substances found in cartilage have had some success as treatments for osteoarthritis. Do they really work? Sometimes. But it takes eight full weeks for the treatment to take effect. If you want to try these pills, you can find them on the open shelf of your pharmacy or in a health food store. But, if there is no improvement after two months, stop. These pills are expensive; they are only worth taking if they work. Good scientific studies mea-suring their worth should be available soon.
- **Capsaicin cream.** The ingredient in chili peppers that gives them their "oomph" is capsaicin. Using a cream with capsaicin extract has been found to reduce arthritic pain by reducing the amount of substance P in your nerve cells. This substance P is responsible for getting messages of pain to your brain; the lower the amount, the lower your pain. If you have high blood pressure, check with your doctor before trying this

cream, and always make sure you wash your hands after using. You don't want to rub your eye with capsaicin. Ouch!

You can get more information on the different types of arthritis from:

**National Institute of Arthritis
and Musculoskeletal and Skin Diseases**
Building 31, Room 4C05
Bethesda, MD 20892
(301) 496-8188
www.niams.nih.gov

The Arthritis Foundation
1330 West Peachtree Street
Atlanta, GA 30309
(800) 283-7800
(404) 872-7100
www.arthritis.org

This ends our "walk up the stairs" of your house. It's time to walk back down, to the very foundation of your body: your bones.

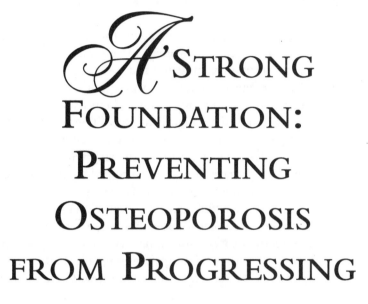

$\mathscr{A}$ STRONG FOUNDATION: PREVENTING OSTEOPOROSIS FROM PROGRESSING

Grow graceful, growing old.
—Anonymous

It wasn't that Greta couldn't get around. She could walk as much as she ever did, to the grocery store, the post office, the pharmacy. Maybe she had to put the seat closer to the steering wheel in her car, but so what? She'd lost a few pounds and looked trim.

But there was something different, or that felt different, anyway, the last few months. Greta would have called it timidity if she'd ever been a fearful person. It was just that she didn't walk with as much forthrightness as before. Her strides weren't as long. Her gait wasn't as steady.

Greta was afraid of falling, and one bright, sunny afternoon, her fear became a reality. She was walking from her apartment house to a boutique down the street; she'd been eyeing a skirt she'd seen in the window. One minute she was walking on the sidewalk, the next, she was on it, her arm twisted underneath her.

Greta was lucky. When a kindly neighbor took her to the emergency room, she learned that she'd fractured her wrist. She'd need to wear a cast for a few weeks, but she should be as good as new. The bruise on her hip and her scraped knee would soon be memories.

But, in spite of the good news, the doctor was concerned. Greta was a 58-year-old woman in reasonably good health. But she'd gone through menopause four years ago and hadn't started any hormone replacement therapy program. She was a tiny woman with a small frame and, although she'd cut back on the fats in her diet, she still enjoyed her nightly martinis. The factor that most gave the emergency room doctor concern was Greta's casual mention that she had to move closer to the steering wheel in her car. That, and the fall itself, gave him a reason to order a bone density study.

It was as the doctor suspected: Greta had osteoporosis. In fact, she'd had it for a while. On one level, Greta was relieved; there was nothing neurological about her unsteady walk—or the fact that she seemed to be "shrinking." But she was now afraid that she'd end up with a "dowager's hump," the bent-over result of osteoporosis a few of her friends exhibited. Greta's family physician was hopeful. He put her on a new medication specifically designed to halt osteoporosis; he also started hormone replacement therapy to restore her estrogen levels. He was confident Greta's condition would get no worse.

Greta took her medicine diligently. She also started doing weight-bearing exercises at her local gym. She made sure she took calcium supplements and drank two glasses of skim milk every day.

There was nothing Greta could do about the loss of bone density she already had, the weakened bones that caused her to fall. But she was determined to do everything right from this moment on. She would make sure that the osteoporosis stopped here and now.

Greta is not alone. Today, 28 million Americans have osteoporosis—and 80% of them are women. Even more sobering: Osteoporosis is the cause behind 1.5 million bone fractures every year, including 300,000 hip fractures and 250,000 wrist fractures.

One out of every two women (and one out of every eight men) will have an osteoporosis-caused fracture within their lives.

But don't run out to buy a cane just yet. Like Greta, there are some things that you can do right now to help prevent osteoporosis—and to stop it from getting worse. You can protect the foundation of your "house" with the right tools.

And that begins with knowledge.

The old saying that oatmeal is good for you because it "sticks to your bones" is not far off. A healthy, hot meal provides the fuel to get your muscles moving—and your muscles surround your bones. Without bones, your muscles would be so much "glop." Your organs would not have a perfect "cocoon" to nestle in; they might get crushed. Your bones are your framework, the strength in your skeleton, the basic foundation of movement.

As we grow up, until about the age of 30, our bones are constantly being "remodeled." Like the house you live in, your old bones are constantly being worn down. But instead of calling in a contractor, your body automatically replaces them with stronger, new bones. This cyclic process is called resorption and formation, and it means that your bones are living, growing tissue. Except for a small amount of the protein collagen, bone is comprised of calcium phosphate. In fact, 99% of the calcium in your body is found in your bones (the other 1% stays in your bloodstream).

This process of bone replacement continues without a hitch for most of us until we reach middle age. At around 30, resorption exceeds formation. That means our old bones are being broken down faster than they can be replaced with new bones. The result? Weaker, more porous bones. Bones with less mineral density. Old bones.

As any aging baby boomer can attest, "old bones" do not necessarily mean bad bones. Some people, men and women, live fracture-free throughout their lives. Their bones might be old, but they have enough strength to last them well through their senior years.

But for many of us, especially post-menopausal women, bone loss reaches a point where fractures occur. These fractures can be very painful and, because of the bone mineral-density loss, bones

BEAM ME UP

Dual Energy X-ray Absorptiometry (DXA) . . . Single Photon Absorptiometry (SPA) . . . Quantitative Computed Tomography. These terms might sound like weapons from the latest Star Trek episode, but in reality, they are very effective diagnostic tools to determine whether or not you have osteoporosis. All the tests are simple, take just minutes, and have no risk. By measuring the bone density in your wrist, hip, and lower spine, doctors can tell if you've lost some of the mineral mass in your bones and if they've begun to weaken.

might not heal properly. Your bones may change shape. This is called osteoporosis and, because you might not realize you have it until you break a bone, it is often called "the silent disease."

*R*ISK TAKERS

Although osteoporosis has been known to strike anyone, at any age, there are some predispositions, some risks, that make some people more prone to the disease than others. These include:

- *Menopause.* It may not be fair, but the loss of estrogen after menopause affects women's bone density. The extra testosterone produced by men helps protect them from bone loss.
- *A small frame.* Petite women are at greater risk, especially the more they age.
- *Height.* Tall people are more likely to injure themselves in a fall because of the increased angle of the fall.
- *Ethnicity.* If you are a Caucasian woman, your risk will be higher than African-Americans or Hispanics.
- *A poor diet.* If you eat foods that are low in calcium and vitamin D, you'll be at a higher risk. Drink your milk!
- *Alcohol consumption.* Excess drinking "leeches" out the calcium from your bones.

- *Smoking.* Here's another reason to quit.
- *A sedentary lifestyle.* If you never get off your couch, your body will pay the price in later life. Exercise builds strong muscles—and bones.
- *A family history.* Yes, if someone close to you had osteoporosis, the risks are higher for you. But they can be abated with a healthy lifestyle.
- *Medications.* If you are taking steroids for arthritis or asthma, diuretics for blood pressure, blood-thinners, or anti-seizure medications for neurological problems, you are at risk for osteoporosis. But to be forewarned is to be forearmed. Have your bone density checked regularly. Get lots of calcium, vitamin D, and exercise. Stop smoking and drink in moderation. Your doctor may place you on one of the new medicines for osteoporosis. (*See below.*)

ℬRING THE BOUNCE BACK IN YOUR BONES

There are many effective treatments out on the market today that really work in halting osteoporosis. Combine them with a healthy lifestyle and you can wave good-bye to weak bones—with gusto! Some of the "strong bone builders" include:

Strong Bone Builder #1: Medical Inroads

All of the medications used for osteoporosis block the breakdown of bone; they are anti-resorptive. You may have heard about Alendronate (Fosamax®) which is usually prescribed for people who have bone density loss (osteoporosis) from any cause. It comes in an easy-to-take, once-a-week pill—giving you stronger bones from the very first week. Side effects may include nausea, stomach cramps, muscle aches, and heartburn. Actonel® is another prescribed medicine for bone density loss.

Scientists have found a new class of medications called Selective Estrogen Receptor Modulators (SERMs) that may also halt bone loss—and prevent it as well. The first SERM to be approved by the FDA is raloxifene (Evista®). It is been found to

TAKE AN ANTIBIOTIC AND CALL ME IN THE MORNING

Studies at the National Institutes of Health have found that minocycline, an antibiotic similar to tetracycline, can increase bone density, enhance bone strength, and slow down the resorption process. In short, minocycline has been found to have the same positive results as estrogen therapy—without the possible side effects.

be successful in treating hipbone loss; it can be a choice for people who can't take estrogen. (*See Strong Bone Builder #2.*) Side effects may include hot flashes and deep vein thrombosis.

For women who cannot take any of the above drugs, Calcitonin (Calcimar®, Miacalcin®) might be a good choice. A natural hormone, this medication has been found to help the pain of bone fractures, as well as help prevent them. Side effects may include flushing, nausea, frequent urination, and skin rashes. It is taken as a nasal spray.

Strong Bone Builder #2: Estrogen

Because the loss of estrogen can bring on osteoporosis, it makes sense that replenishing the hormone in your body will help prevent it. Estrogen replacement helps increase your bone density, keep your bones stronger, and helps prevent bone loss. Researchers aren't sure why estrogen plays such a strong role in bone formation, but they are certain that it does. Because estrogen, taken alone, can increase the risk of uterine cancer, hormone replacement therapy usually involves taking a combination of both estrogen and progesterone. See your doctor to see if you are a good candidate for this treatment. (*See Chapter Six for details on menopause and hormone replacement therapy.*)

Strong Bone Builder #3: Calcium Supplements

The proof is in: calcium, found in milk and other dairy products, will help prevent osteoporosis. Calcium is not only necessary for bone health, but also for healthy hearts, muscles, blood clotting, and nerves as well.

If you don't get enough calcium in your diet or in a supplement, your body will take it from your bones to ensure these other systems get what they need.

You can find calcium in:

- Milk products, such as skim or low-fat milk, yogurt, and ice cream
- Cheese, including cottage cheese, cheddar, and Swiss cheese
- Fruits and vegetables, especially broccoli, oranges, figs, and beans
- Fish (especially sardines) and shellfish
- Tofu and other soy products

Most women don't get enough of these foods and a calcium supplement will help ensure you are getting enough calcium. Citrated calcium, such as Citracel® or Tums® are better absorbed. This is one situation in which you want to be cautious about generics since their absorption from the gastrointestinal tract may vary greatly; it's more difficult to keep track of generics as opposed to brand names. Physicians suggest taking 1200–1500 mg. of calcium a day, usually in combination with vitamin D. (Too much calcium can lead to kidney stones so have your doctor periodically check your blood calcium level.)

Strong Bone Builders #4: Exercise

Lift those weights and tote that barge. It might sound like slavery, but, in reality, the exercise you do now will set you free. Studies have found that exercise, in particular weight-bearing exercise, can reduce the risk of osteoporosis in women. Why? This type of exercise helps maintain bone mass which, in turn, keeps your

SWIM ON

There's more to swimming than a relaxing Sunday afternoon in the summertime. Water exercise is great for bones; the resistance of water works as well as weight-bearing exercises in the gym—at least that's what a study in Japan discovered. A year after beginning a water aerobics class 45 minutes once a week, 35 women had increased their bone density.

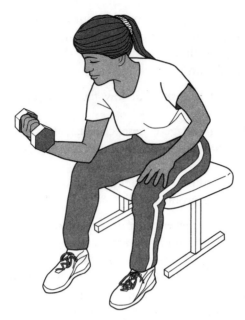

Figure 9–1 Bicep Curl

bones and muscles strong. Most local health clubs have weight rooms and trainers who will show you how to use the machines free of charge. You can also invest in resistance machines for your home gym. A set of weights is a good investment. They are inexpensive, easy to use, and you can purchase them at any sporting goods store. Adjustable weights are a good choice because you can attach more pounds as you get stronger. There are sets that contain 3-, 5-, and 8-pound weights—all in one.

Here are two strength-building exercises to get you going:

Bicep Curl

1. Sit up in a chair, feet flat on the floor. Hold the weight in your right hand, palm up. Bend your right arm and rest it on your right thigh.
2. Move your right arm down for a count of four.
3. Move your arm back up for a count of two.
4. Try to work up to 15 repetitions. Take a break for a few minutes, then repeat 15 times again.
5. Hold the weight in your left hand and repeat the entire exercise on your left arm.

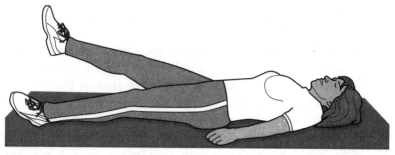

Figure 9–1   Leg extension

Leg Extension

1. Lie down on an exercise mat or towel, face up.
2. Keeping your head, chest, torso, and arms on the mat, slowly lift only one leg up into the air, raising it as high as it can go (without pain!) Keep the other leg flat on the mat.
3. Hold for a count of two.
4. Release. Move your leg back into place at a count of four.
5. Try to do 15 repetitions with one leg. Wait a few minutes, then repeat.
6. Do the entire exercise, including the "rest stop," with the other leg.

You can find more strength-training exercises in your bookstore or library, or contact the:

American Dietetic Association
216 West Jackson Boulevard
Chicago, IL 60606
(312) 899-0040
www.eatright.org

Strong Bone Builders #5: Preventing Falls and Fractures

One of the best ways to avoid falling and breaking a wrist or a hip is to "fall proof" your home. Some suggestions:

- Use the handrail when walking up and down your stairs.
- Stay clear of just-cleaned floors. They can be slippery.
- Take a cue from your grocery store and purchase a "reacher." These tools can help you get something from a high shelf —

or from the floor—without having to balance precariously on a chair or shaky knees.

- Let there be light, strong light, in every room of your house. It's always better to see a misplaced toy or an electric cord first. Make sure you have light switches at both the top and the bottom of the stairs.
- Keep your home free of clutter. Boxes, papers, and objects can literally trip you up.
- Make your bathroom safe with grab bars in the tub, nonskid mats in the shower, tacked-down carpets on the floor, and a nightlight that's always on.
- Use skid-proof backing on all throw rugs. Use self-adhesive strips to keep rugs in place. Better yet: get rid of tricky throw rugs altogether!

These are all the ingredients you need for a strong foundation in your "home." For more information, contact:

National Osteoporosis Foundation (NOF)
1232 22nd Street, NW
Washington, DC 20037-1292
1-202-223-2226
www.nof.org

**National Resource Center on Osteoporosis
and Related Diseases**
1-800-624-BONE (2663)
(202) 223-0344 (TTY)
www.osteo.org

Now that our foundation is in place, we can move on to other crucial areas of your home. Nothing is more illuminating than windows. Let's go on to the windows in your house—and your eyes which see through them.

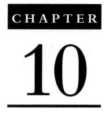

WINDOWS OF THE SOUL: VISION LOSS

To be seventy years young is sometimes far more cheerful and hopeful than to be forty years old.
—Oliver Wendell Holmes, Jr.

Barbara made her living by the numbers. Literally. She was an accountant, and rows of figures and a calculator were her constant companions. She might have had eyestrain every so often, after hours looking at her computer screen, but she just chalked it up to the hazards of her job.

In fact, Barbara never gave her eyes much thought. She might rub them when she was tired. She might use drops if they were dry and itchy from the smog. She sometimes looked at her eyelids, becoming droopy with age, and thought about cosmetic surgery. But that was all. Like breathing or scratching an itch, her eyes were there, an unconscious part of her.

But that was before her vision became a bit blurry, before she had difficulty reading a paperback book at night, before she had trouble reading a menu in a dim restaurant. And that was *with* her glasses on!

Although somewhat disconcerted, Barbara chalked it up to old age. After all, she wasn't a kid anymore. She was in her late sixties, and everyone's eyes got weaker as they aged.

All that changed when Barbara found it hard to read her numbers. There she was, sunlight streaming through her office windows, halogen lights up high, and she still couldn't read the fine print. Barbara was scared; she felt too young to retire. And what could she do without her precious eyesight. . . .

Barbara made an appointment with her ophthalmologist that same day. The doctor told her what she already knew: her eyes had grown worse. But what she hadn't known was that she had developed a cataract in her left eye; it was clouding her vision.

"Am I going blind?" she asked, suddenly terrified of the future. The doctor smiled. Not by a long shot. In today's world, cataract surgery can be performed on an outpatient basis; it is one of the most common surgeries, with over 500,000 performed every year. Highly-refined modern surgical techniques using ultrasound energy and miniature implanted lenses make it a routine procedure, practically painless. Although Barbara would have to wear an eye patch overnight, her eyesight would improve very rapidly after surgery, perhaps even by the next day.

The ophthalmologist recommended that Barbara get a pair of sunglasses that blocked both UVA and UVB (ultraviolet) rays. She suggested that for added protection she wear a hat with a visor when she went out in the sun. And she told her to start eating more fruits and vegetables. The antioxidants in these foods would keep her eyes strong.

Barbara took her doctor's advice. No longer would she take her eyes for granted. Today she still does part-time accounting work, but she spends most of her time in her sunroom, sewing needlepoint pillows, pictures, and eyeglass cases for her family and friends. You can also find her reading the latest best-seller in the hammock in her backyard, sun visor and sunglasses in place.

If you are like Barbara and take your eyes for granted, don't feel bad. Most people do—until something goes wrong. It's sort of like that old adage, "If it isn't broken, don't fix it." If your house is in good condition, why bother doing touch-ups?

But by taking care of things before they are broken, ensuring that your foundation stays strong, your roof stays solid, and your windows stay clean, you'll get much more joy out of your house.

Similarly, by taking care of your eyes now, before they worsen with age, you will find that they'll take you far into the years to come. And, even if you, like Barbara, have been diagnosed with an eye problem, you can often stop it from getting worse.

Before you can change things, however, you need to know exactly where to "look." You need to know *how* you see what you see.

THE EYES HAVE IT

The invention of the camera didn't materialize out of thin air. It very much imitates your eyes. And if you think of those eyes as a one-click camera, you can get a good idea of how you see:

1. *First, you focus.* Imagine the eyeball being a camera. Light from outside "hits" the cornea, then the lens. The iris, in the center of the eye, adjusts the amount of light that enters your eye via the pupil; small ciliary muscles shape the lens and help focus what you are seeing.

2. *Then you see.* The retina in the back of the eye is comprised of two types of cells: cones and rods—3 million cones and 100 million rods, to be exact. Cones, with their three pigments, enable you to see color. The rods help you see in dim light; they are responsible for black and white. Like an actual camera, the image that hits the back of the eye is actually backwards and upside down from the one we actually see.

3. *Always leave room for interpretation.* Once the rods and cones get their "hits" of light from the front of the eye, they are able to do the job they were "born" to do: transfer the ray of light into nerve signals—which travel, via the optic nerve, back to the brain. Here, in the occipital lobe at the back of the brain, is where we first "see" an image. From the occipital lobe, the information we've "seen" is sent to other parts of the brain, specifically the parietal and temporal lobes (*see Chapter Four for details on the brain and the rest of the nervous system*). In the parietal and temporal lobes, the original visual image is now translated, activated, and linked to memories already stored. Now you not only can see, but also perceive your version of reality. Now you can "know" that that furry object with the long claws is a cat.

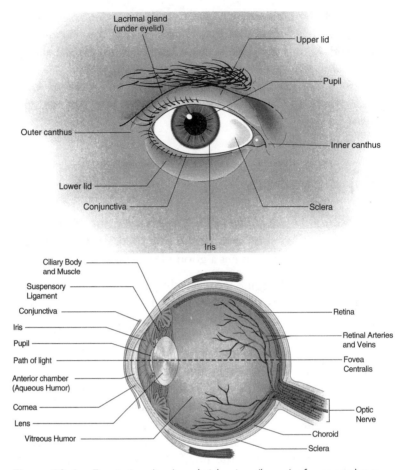

Figure 10–1   Front view (top) and side view (lower) of a normal eye.

As you age, this process of seeing will continue—but the light rays that hit your eye may become distorted; the light might not be able to effectively enter your cornea; the retina might not be able to decipher the rays of light. Certain diseases can also cause vision problems. Atherosclerosis can cause a stroke in the retina or brain and subsequent loss of vision. Macular degeneration (*discussed in the next section*) can affect the most sensitive part of the retina and lead to loss of central vision. Diabetes can cause bleeding and damage in your retina.

Although many people continue to have excellent eyesight well into their 80s, some do develop certain age-related eye conditions. Some of these are easily fixed; others can be stopped before they get any worse. Like the windows in your home, the

"EYE" SEE

You probably know that 20/20 vision is normal, but did you ever wonder what these numbers actually mean? The first number refers to how many feet away you are from the numbers on the eye chart in your doctor's office. The second number tells you the distance at which a person with normal vision can see the eye chart clearly. In other words, if your vision was 20/40, what you can see from 20 feet a person with normal vision could see from 40 feet.

If your eye doctor diagnoses astigmatism, you have a cornea that's slightly oval instead of being perfectly round. You might have blurry vision.

Whatever the reason you need to wear glasses, today's laser refractive surgery may correct your condition. Ask your doctor if you are a good candidate for the procedure. Remember, however, that although people are rushing to have this done, it is a relatively new procedure and its long-term effects are not yet completely known. There are occasional side effects that can permanently alter your vision. Think it through. Talk to your doctor. Make sure it's the right choice for you.

best views are from those panes that are kept clean, fixed when broken, and continually maintained.

Let's go over some of the eye problems you may encounter as you age.

THE BIG MAC: MACULAR DEGENERATION

There's more to the retina "than meets the eye." In addition to rods and cones, your retina contains a small 1/16 inch spot called the macula. This minute area holds more receptors than any other area of the eyeball. It is responsible for straight-ahead, focused

vision. The macula enables you to watch TV, to read, to drive a car, sew, or do close work.

As you get older, the macula may become scarred. Yellow deposits develop beneath it, in the blood vessels, creating degeneration of the nerve tissue. The result is age-related macular degeneration (ARMD). You might find the lines on a page beginning to waver; your central field of vision isn't as sharp; you experience blank spots.

If any of these symptoms sounds familiar, you're in good company. Approximately 13 million Americans have ARMD—usually after the age of 55.

Although macular degeneration can't be reversed, there are some things you can do to stop it from getting worse:

- *See your ophthalmologist.* Getting a yearly eye exam is crucial at any age, but particularly as you get older. Your doctor can determine if there has been any macular degeneration by means of a harmless procedure—fluorescein angiography—that takes photographs of your retina. In some cases, laser surgery can halt the disease's progression.
- *Eat your eggs.* Studies have found that the protein in the yolks of eggs can actually halt macular degeneration. Doctors recommend eating three eggs a week.
- *Think antioxidant.* The latest research shows that antioxidants, those vitamins and minerals that fight age-related disease in your body and on your skin, also help keep the blood vessels in your retina potent. Most multivitamins are rich in antioxidants such as vitamin C, E, beta-carotene, zinc, and selenium. Check with your doctor about the possibility of increasing the doses if you have macular degeneration.

$\mathcal{C}$ATARACT CONTACT

It is a fact of life: Live long enough and you will develop a cataract in your eye. This might not happen until well into your 90s, but cataracts—an opaque clouding of the lens of the eye that can lead to blurry vision and, ultimately, blindness—is a symptom of aging.

The proteins that make up the composition of your eye's lens start out clear. But over time, as chemicals shift and change, the proteins become cloudy and a cataract forms. If you have any of the following symptoms, see your ophthalmologist as soon as possible:

- Blurry vision
- A blinding glare when looking at automobile headlights
- Seeing halos around street lamps
- Troubled night vision
- Short-term improved nearsightedness. Some people develop cataracts at the center (or nucleus) of the eye, which creates a slight swelling in the lens. This swelling, in turn, can help your eyes focus—so much so that you might not need your reading glasses! But it won't last.

Although cataracts are a normal part of the aging process, certain things can hurry them along, including:

- *Too much sunlight.* Overexposure to ultraviolet B (UVB) rays can change the chemical makeup of the proteins in your eyes.
- *Smoking.* Yet another reason to quit!
- Air pollution and smog.
- *Too much alcohol.* Drinking, driving—and reading—don't mix.
- *Glaucoma.* Sometimes cataracts can be a side effect of this other age-related eye condition. (*See the next section for information on glaucoma.*)

The good news is that cataracts are treated with minimal interruption of your normal activities via outpatient surgery

IF THE EYEGLASSES FIT, DON'T NECESSARILY WEAR THEM

You might think you're doing right by your eyes if you purchase a pair of dark-tinted sunglasses. But fashion statements aside, your misty grey or exotic brown sunglasses might not be UVB-protected—which can actually increase your risk of getting a cataract. Without UVB protection, the pupils of your eyes widen to adjust to the darkness of the glass tint— which will just let more UVB rays in! Make sure the next pair of sunglasses you buy are both UVA- and UVB-protected. Ask. Read the labels.

under local anesthesia. The surgeon makes a small incision at the edge of the cornea using an ultrasonic needle called a Phaco-Emulsifier. The cloudy lens is removed through the incision and replaced with a clear plastic lens. You may not even need stitches!

In the United States alone, 500,000 cataract operations are performed every year. What's more: Complications are rare, and vision is improved to the maximum capability of the eye.

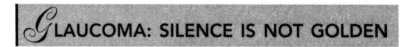

GLAUCOMA: SILENCE IS NOT GOLDEN

Physicians have called glaucoma "the sneak thief in the night" because it can silently rob you of your sight. There are usually no symptoms—until the disease is advanced. You might find that you get sudden intense headaches; your vision might get blurry; you might see "rainbows" around street lamps; you might need stronger glasses. Eventually, your side, or peripheral vision, will diminish, and you'll see black spots instead of an image.

Although these symptoms are sobering and require an immediate visit to the ophthalmologist, it's important to remember that glaucoma can be treated. A disease that affects most people in middle age, it may have a genetic root: one out of every five people who gets glaucoma has a family history of the disease. Glaucoma may also occur in people who have diabetes.

In order to understand what glaucoma is, you need to know some basic eye facts: Your eye is nourished internally by aqueous humor, a water-based liquid that is continuously replenished. As new fluid is created by specialized secretory cells in the eye, the "old," excess fluid is drained out of the eye through a filter area called the trabecular meshwork located at the junction of the cornea and the iris. This filtered fluid then enters the bloodstream via a collection channel called Schlemm's canal.

When the draining of excess fluid slows down, due to aging-related changes in drainage duct angles, pressure may build up. New fluid continues to be produced—and the excess fluid has nowhere to go. This gradual build-up is called chronic, or open-angle, glaucoma. It is the most common form of the disease in older patients.

Sometimes, anatomy places the iris so close to the cornea ("at narrow angles") that the drainage area can be blocked by a dilating

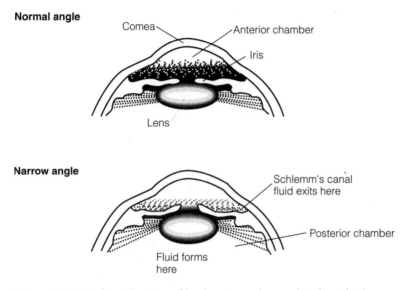

Normal angle

Comea — Anterior chamber

Iris

Lens

Narrow angle

Schlemm's canal fluid exits here

Posterior chamber

Fluid forms here

Figure 10–2 The side view of both a normal eye, detailing the lens, iris, cornea, drainage angle, and Schlemm's canal, and a side view of the same eye with glaucoma

pupil. The pressure in the eye then rises fast and furious. This is called acute glaucoma and can occur at any age. Pain and foggy vision occur rapidly.

Unless the excess fluid is decreased through medication, the use of lasers, or surgery, the built-up, pent-up, pressure eventually damages the optic nerve and sight is affected.

No one knows exactly why some people get glaucoma—and others get away scot-free. Some risk factors may include:

- *Certain medications.* Antidepressants, hypertension pills, and corticosteroids may cause increased pressure.
- *Collagen metabolism.* The same substance that keeps your skin looking smooth can also keep your eyesight keen. If this protein, abundant in the tissues of the eye, breaks down, it can affect fluid drainage and eye strength.

Your ophthalmologist can determine if you have glaucoma by using a complex-sounding tool called an applanation tonometer, which measures the pressure inside your eye. Your optometrist will use an air-puff tonometer—and if you've ever had this test, you'll remember it. A puff of air is literally blown into your eye to measure pressure.

If your ophthalmologist detects glaucoma in your eye, he may prescribe one of the following:

- *Beta-blocker eye drops.* These names read like an alien language: timolol, betaxolol, and bunolol. But they can do the trick in reducing fluid production in your eyes and increasing outflow. But, as always, there may be side effects. These may include asthma, slower heart rate, depression, and possible sexual dysfunction.
- *Carbonic anhydrase inhibitors.* These come in pill form and work on slowing down fluid production in the eye. Possible side effects can include stomach pain and tingling in the hands or feet. These are rarely used today, and have been replaced by the eyedrop preparations Azopt® and Cosopt®.
- *Prostaglandin inhibitors.* These new drugs promote increased outflow of the fluid and only need to be used once a day. Their only side effect? They may darken a light-colored iris.
- *Trabeculoplasty laser surgery.* If medication doesn't seem to work, or if the side effects are too uncomfortable, your doctor may suggest surgery. Here, laser beams hit the angle of the drainage duct, creating more space for fluid to drain.
- *Trabeculectomy.* This more involved procedure is used when other means are unsuccessful, or if the glaucoma is far advanced. In this surgery, an artifical replacement drainage canal, including new angles, is actually constructed in your eye.

If you've begun to develop some problems with your eyes— some "cloudy windows," all is not lost. The eyes are one of the hardiest organs in your body; they can stand up to a lot of stress. Glaucoma is highly treatable and the functional loss of vision in glaucoma is rare these days. There have also been tremendous advances in eye surgery procedures—and there are several preventative measures you can take right now to avoid your eyes worsening.

Here are some "Eye Advantages" you can use right now:

Eye Advantage #1: Contact Cleanliness

It's easy to take your contact lenses for granted, especially if you've worn them for many, many years. Perhaps you forget to disinfect them one night. Maybe you stopped using your enzyme cleaner for a while. Or maybe you haven't gotten a new pair in more than two years. Whatever the reason, stop! Take care of your contacts.

Clean them daily. Respect them as if they were your eyes. New disposable lenses have eliminated many of these problems—but only if you use them properly!

Eye Advantage #2: Avoid Eyestrain

This might sound simpler than it really is. You might know to give your eyes a rest when they start to burn and blink after close work. But did you know that the dim light illuminating your computer might be contributing to your eyestrain? Or that the small print in the contract really is too small? Keep a magnifying glass available. Take advantage of both high-intensity spotlights and contrast lighting that gets rid of shadows and glare. As we age, it is more difficult to see in full sunlight or under fluorescent lights. Avoid glare and try to create contrasts with lighting. Opt for hardcover books instead of impossible-to-read paperbacks. A good way to rest your eyes: close them. Take a five-minute break and put moistened cotton balls or tea bags over your eyelids. Aahh. Take a few minutes now and your future will reap the rewards.

Eye Advantage #3: Think Shade

Sunlight might feel wonderful on your skin, but give your eyes a break. Avoid harmful, eye-damaging UVA and UVB rays by

THE HANG-DOG LOOK

Your longing to erase those droopy eyelids may be more than vanity. Your eyelids protect your eyes and control light; they dispense tears with every blink. But, as you age, the skin of your eyelids loses its elasticity. The result is droopy eyelids which can make seeing difficult. Surgery can correct the problem—and, as an added benefit, "blink" back the years.

Another eyelid conditions that may occur with age is blepharitis, which is red, inflamed eyelids—and another reason to think of surgery.

wearing proper sunglasses, sunscreen, and hats with rims. Who knows? You just might be mistaken for your favorite movie star!

Eye Advantage #4: Eat Your Spinach

And carrots, oranges, and all other fruits and vegetables. They are chock full of antioxidants, those eye-loving vitamins and minerals that help fight the damage caused by aging. In fact, a Harvard University study found that women who ate five servings of spinach a week cut their risk of cataracts by 47%. The ongoing Nurses Health Study found that women who took between 400 and 700 mg of vitamin C every day for more than 10 years reduced the risk of developing cataracts by 80%.

Other eye-rich supplements include the phytonutrients. These plant chemicals are full of antioxidants that keep eyes strong. You'll find them in foods such as blueberries and grapes. Supplements that contain these "super" ingredients include lycopene, bilberry, lutein, and zeaxanthin.

SURGERY BY ANY OTHER NAME

It's called lasik, and it's the hottest new surgery available. It can create near perfect vision in people who have been nearsighted or farsighted all their lives.

Performed on an outpatient basis, this relatively pain-free procedure uses a computer-guided knife to slice the cornea and lift up its outer layer. The laser reshapes the cornea. The flap is then closed, and near-perfect vision is created.

Side effects can include a temporary problem seeing at night, seeing halos around lights, headaches, and, in some cases, overcorrected vision, or farsightedness. It is also expensive.

Is lasik for you? The early success rate is astonishingly high. People who have always worn thick glasses, or who've just started to wear bifocals, can toss them in the garbage. But check with your doctor. Learn as much as you can, and be aware that we still do not know the long-term effects.

Eye Advantage #5: Check Up Smarts

Seeing is believing and the best way to ensure your sight stays strong is to "see" your eye doctor once a year—especially as you approach middle age. Eye problems, as with any other condition, are always best treated in the early stages. Having a yearly vision test is the only way to guarantee early detection.

For more information about your eyes, investigate:

American Academy of Ophthalmology
P. O. Box 7424
San Francisco, CA   94120
(415) 561-8500
(415) 561-8567 (fax)
www.eyenet.org/

National Eye Institute
2020 Vision Place
Bethesda, MD 20892
(301) 496-5248
(301) 402-1065 (fax)
www.nei.nih.gov

It's time now to turn away from the windows of your house—and walk outside to your back porch. Listen to the sounds of summer, and learn how your hearing can be affected as you age.

11

$\mathcal{S}$OUNDS OF SUMMER ON THE BACK PORCH: HEARING LOSS

We are all here for a spell; get all the good laughs you can.
—Will Rogers

Emily used to play this game: When she and her friends were about 10 years old and learning about the five senses in school, they'd ask themselves which sense would be the worst to lose. It changed almost daily. Sometimes it was sight, sometimes touch. Other times it was taste. But Emily never varied in her idea of hell: the loss of hearing.

Emily's father played violin for the New York Philharmonic, one of the most famous orchestras in the world. Her mother had been an opera singer. And, since she was five, Emily had been playing a musical instrument. Music was in her life; it surrounded her. It was her life.

Although Emily never became the concert pianist she'd once dreamed of being, she had still gained a reputation as one of the most renowned authorities on music theory. She taught music at a prestigious Ivy League school, and she had one of the most extensive collections of rare recordings in the world.

Emily's days and nights were filled with music. Anyone, a friend, a contractor, the mailman, could come to her house any time of the day or night and if she was home, there'd be music playing.

But, lately, even the neighbors down the block could hear the music. Emily had begun to play her CDs louder and louder. In school, students noticed she needed them to ask the same questions more than once. Even her friends, on a dinner out, would notice that she didn't join in the conversation too much.

One night, a colleague from the university rang her bell. They had made plans to go to a nearby concert. There was no answer. Emily's friend rang it again. Still nothing. He peered into the bay window near the door. Emily was sitting on a sofa, her reading lamp on. She was reading and sipping a glass of wine as she turned the pages.

Emily's friend knocked on the window. She still didn't turn around. Her friend was sure it was because of the music. Perhaps it was on so loudly that she couldn't hear the doorbell. He took out his cell phone and dialed Emily's number. He heard it ring . . . and ring. Emily continued to read and sip her wine.

Just when he was about to give up in frustration, Emily glanced up from her book and looked out the window. She saw her friend and nearly dropped her glass. She ran to the door.

Emily's friend was furious—and worried. He stomped into the house, ready to turn off her CD player, when he stopped cold. The house was silent. Quiet. There was no music on.

But Emily still hadn't heard the doorbell. The knock on the window. The phone. She hadn't known her friend had been trying to get her attention for almost half an hour.

Emily finally had to face what she'd been ignoring and rationalizing away for months: She was losing her sense of sound. Emily had a hearing loss—and it was getting worse.

At first, Emily was inconsolable. She began to withdraw from her friends and family. She took a leave of absence from the university. She became irritable, her usual good nature disappearing. But, eventually, Emily learned to accept what she couldn't change—and to use whatever tools were available to help her hear.

Emily had presbycusis, the most common type of hearing loss in the elderly—a slow, decreasing progression as the inner ear changes. Although she couldn't do anything about her declining condition, she was able to get a new state-of-the-art hearing aid that was not only light and practically invisible, but also music to her ears. She could hear!

It wasn't perfect. There were times, in restaurants, when conversation sounded like a low din. There were times when she couldn't hear certain instruments during a quiet symphony movement. But, in most cases, Emily managed just fine. She purchased a loud bell for her phone and another one for her door. She used earphones to listen to her music. She made sure her hearing aid was working properly, especially before class. And she visited her doctor frequently to make sure that wax didn't build up in her ears—which would only exacerbate her condition.

All in all, Emily was leading a fine life. She considered herself very lucky indeed—despite the loss of one of her senses. In fact, you might say that she "came to her senses" at last.

Emily's career path might be less than ordinary, but her condition is more common than you might think. If you have just celebrated your 65th birthday, it's possible that you will join the more than 33% of all Americans who have some sort of hearing loss. And, if you are over 85, the figure grows to 50% the population.

But there is hearing loss—and there is hearing loss. There are many different types of loss and many different levels *within* those losses. Perhaps you, like Emily, cannot hear the doorbell. Or maybe you just have problems with one-on-one conversation. Or you could miss words in a play, or a musical riff here and there.

The aging person with a hearing problem is almost a cliché. The gray-haired woman blaring her television so she can watch her game shows. The balding man who nods his head when you ask him a question. The husband who asks you to stop using the vacuum cleaner because it is so loud that he cannot hear himself think.

Unfortunately, this oh-so-common condition creates an energy of its own—one that can spiral down into depression and isolation. When people cannot hear, they get embarrassed and flustered. Rather than ask to have something repeated over and over again, they'll withdraw. They don't want to be a burden. But, with this withdrawal, can come irritability, pain, and paranoia. You start to think that people are mumbling on purpose! Maybe they're talking about you!

It doesn't have to be this way. Let's look at the ear, an organ of amazing complexity, and learn about hearing—and the loss of it.

𝒟ID YOU HEAR THAT?

Believe it or not, the outer ear, the part of your ear that you show the world (or cover up) has almost no function, except to gather sound. Its shape helps to bring sound waves into the ear canal.

Sound enters the ear canal and strikes the eardrum, or the tympanic membrane. As the eardrum vibrates, it causes a bone in the middle ear called the malleus, as well as two other bones linked to it—the incus and the stapes—to move. These three bones are connected to each other; the eardrum and malleus movement is easily transmitted to the incus and the stapes (the smallest bone in the body). Because the stapes is positioned over the inner ear fluids, when it vibrates these fluids move as well.

SWIMMING WITH SHARKS

Swimming laps might be a great form of exercise, but it can be too much of a good thing. If your ears get clogged with water from the pool or lake, you might find yourself with ear pain and temporary hearing loss.

To avoid "swimmer's ear":

Place several drops of a mixture of equal parts alcohol and white vinegar in your ear. The alcohol helps to eliminate the water in the ear canal while the vinegar leaves an acidic environment which prevents bacterial and fungal infections. You can also use a product like Swim-Ear®, an over-the-counter preparation which performs like the alcohol/white vinegar mixture.

Avoid cleaning your ears the day before you plan on swimming. The wax you remove protects your ear from water seeping in.

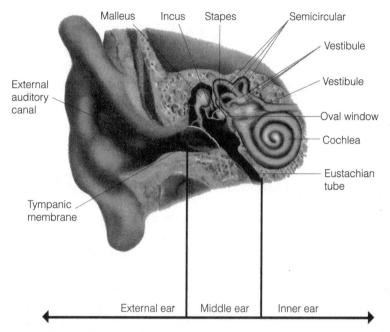

Figure 11–1   Drawing of the outer, middle, and inner ear

The middle ear is made up of the same mucus membranes that line your sinuses and nasal passageway—and it is just as vulnerable to colds, flus, and allergies. This is why your ears get clogged up and achy, adding to your distress when you're sick.

Think of the third and final portion of the ear as the "inner sanctum," the place where a rock concert, a scream, a sigh, a laugh, is transported to the auditory nerve and, eventually, to the brain for interpretation. Just as the malleus, incus, and stapes look like an anvil, a hammer, and stirrups, the main portion of the inner ear—the cochlea—looks like something else, too: a snail. It is filled with fluid and contains thousands of tiny hair cells which respond to different frequencies of sound. When sound enters the inner ear, fluid movement bends the tiny hair cells. This mechanical bending changes that voice, noise, or sweet music from a sound wave to an electrical impulse which move along the hearing nerve to the brain.

The inner ear is also responsible for your balance. Thanks to the labyrinth, a series of semicircular canals, shaped liked doughnuts and filled with fluid, you are able to avoid getting dizzy when you move. This liquidy substance helps keep an image stable on your retina—even when you shake your head.

As difficult as it is to imagine so many different organs in one small ear, there are still two more that "roar." These are the otolith organs, your two sentinels of balance. When you move your head, the otoliths tell your brain that you're on the go—and in what direction you're bound.

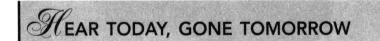 HEAR TODAY, GONE TOMORROW

For such a complicated, delicate system, the ears work amazingly well. For many people throughout their lives, sound is a sense with staying power. Yes, as with any portion of your house, you might lose some subtlety, some nuance, of sound and frequency as time passes—just as rocking chairs and screen doors become slightly worn from use. However, on the whole, your ability to hear is, well, as clear as a bell—and as strong as a memory of the sounds of a long-ago summer on your back porch.

But things can happen, especially over time. If you experience any of the following symptoms, you might have some hearing loss—and you should make an appointment with your doctor for a hearing test:

- It's difficult to understand what people are saying.
- People sound as if they are mumbling or slurring their words, especially in crowds.
- You find some sounds so irritating and loud that they hurt your ears.
- You've stopped going out to dinner or the movies because you can't clearly hear what's going on—so you don't enjoy yourself.
- There's a ringing or hissing sound in your ear—and it's not the phone, the teapot, or the radiator.

Any of these red flags signals a loss of hearing. But what about the reasons behind the inability to decipher sound? What about the why of hearing loss?

The reasons behind hearing problems, like ears themselves, come in all shapes and sizes. Since you need to be exposed to sound in the first place to hear it, we call the reasons behind hearing loss **EXPOSURE**, and there's a factor for each letter in the word:

- *E is for elementary genetics*, the role heredity and DNA arrangement play in the construction of your ear and your ability to hear. A condition called otosclerosis, for example, which prevents the stapes bone from vibrating in the middle ear, is inherited.

- *X-ternals* include acts of God, fate, an accident that leaves you with an inner ear injury. A ruptured eardrum or dislocation of the bone can also cause hearing problems.

- *P is for pills*, the medications you may get in a hospital setting or those your doctor may prescribe. Certain antibiotics, high blood pressure diuretics, quinine, and high doses of aspirin (at least 8–12 a day for a period of time) can affect your hearing.

- *Overkill* can hurt your ears—such as in listening to loud music when you were in your teens, working on a job that entails unrelenting noise, or regularly participating in activities, like hunting and snowmobiling, that go bang (with a bang!).

- *Strokes* can leave you with hearing loss, depending on the area of the brain that is affected.

- *U is when you are under attack* from germs, bacteria, or a virus. Mucus membranes in your middle ear get clogged, resulting in fluid in the middle ear. Other infections may affect the inner ear, causing loss of its hair cells.

- *R is for respiratory and heart conditions.* Respiratory infections can also result in middle ear infections—and vascular disease, such as atherosclerosis and high blood pressure, can lead to stroke and hearing loss.

- *E stands for the erosion of youth.* Age, in particular, affects the tiny hair cells in your inner ear. These hairs eventually fall away and your ability to determine sound frequency deteriorates. This is largely controlled by our genetic makeup.

𝒽EAR SAY: THE DIFFERENT TYPES OF HEARING LOSS

EXPOSURE means just that: your hearing has been affected by a variety of factors, either in your genes or your environment. But the way that exposure is expressed can take several different forms. Here are the most common "ear rings," or hearing problems, that can affect "your home":

EAR JET LAG

It's not an old myth: If you fly with a cold, you can hurt your ears. The condition is called aerotitis media, or barotrauma, and it means that your eardrums have been pushed in because of air pressure changes on landing. If you are stuffed up, no air can get to the middle ear—preventing the rebalancing of the pressure.

If you have to fly with a cold, here are some tips:

Nasal decongestants work. Use one before and after your trip. Spray each nostril shortly before take off and after landing.

Chew gum! It helps open the eustachian tube and allow passage of air into the middle ear.

Look silly: Take a deep breath through your mouth, then hold your nose. Close your mouth and, at the same time, put your tongue on the roof of your mouth. Swallow. This will allow air to go through the eustachian tube to the middle ear, and your ears will unclog.

Ear Ring #1: Presbycusis

Remember those tiny hair cells in the inner ear? Their slow deterioration over time is called presbycusis, and it is the most common hearing problem in people over 50. The loss is so slow, however, that it may never get any worse than missing a word or two in conversation. Just as people get gray hair at different rates, the effects of presbycusis may vary.

Ear Ring #2: Conductive Hearing Loss

This is a loss of transportation, in carrying sound from the ear canal through to the inner ear. When this passageway gets blocked—whether it's due to excess wax, an accidental rupture of the eardrum, fluid or a growth in the middle ear, or an inability of one of the bones in the middle ear to vibrate—sound cannot be transmitted to the inner ear's hair cells. This means that the sound is never actually "heard" or hauled onto the auditory nerve for transport—and interpretation in—the brain.

Ear Ring #3: Sensorineural Hearing Loss

While conductive hearing loss usually subsides with proper medical or surgical care, sensorineural hearing loss is another matter. Here, damage occurs in either the inner ear or in the auditory nerve leading up to the brain. Although this hearing problem can be genetic, it can also be the result of exposure to loud sounds, stroke, head and ear injury, or as a reaction to certain medications.

For many aging baby boomers, hearing loss may be a combination of both conductive and sensorineural problems. A hearing aid can help—as can a more quiet environment that doesn't tax your ears.

Ear Ring #4: Tinnitus

Think of a constant ringing or buzzing in your ears and you'll get an idea of the irritation of tinnitus. This conditions appears in about 30 percent of people over 50, and it can sometimes disappear spontaneously. In fact, some people have tinnitus and aren't even aware of it. They take the background noise for granted; it's just part of the white noise of life, along with traffic, restaurant chatter, or static on the radio.

Tinnitus may be caused by earwax buildup, middle ear problems (such as infection), loss of hair cells in the inner ear, or as a reaction to certain medications.

Tinnitus can occur concurrently with problems in the balance portion of the inner ear. It can also pulsate, like your heart beat, if vascular problems are involved. Although further evaluation is recommended if your tinnitus occurs in only one ear, most types are nothing to worry about.

Ear Ring #5: Meniere's Disease

Yes, there was a Dr. Meniere, a French physician to be exact, who lived in the 18th century and who first diagnosed this condition as vertigo. Remember those doughnut-like balance tubes filled with fluid in the inner ear? (*See Figure 11–1 on page 157.*) When the inner ear liquid builds up, either from hereditary factors, trauma, or a too-salty diet, the excess fluid causes a loss of balance. You might also experience hearing loss, tinnitus, nausea, and dizziness. Recurring bouts of the disease can lead to permanent hearing loss, but you can help manage Meniere's with a salt-restrictive

diet, doctor-prescribed diuretics, a rehabilitation program with special exercises, and a healthy lifestyle that includes coping better with stress and quitting smoking.

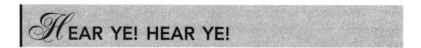 EAR YE! HEAR YE!

First things first. If you believe you are experiencing hearing loss, you should pick up the phone and call a doctor, either your family physician, an otologist, or a hearing care provider who deals specifically with the ears.

You'll most likely need to take a hearing test called an audiogram. You enter a soundproof booth, but instead of hoping to win a million dollars in a quiz show, you'll don earphones and listen to sounds. The technician on the other side of the booth regulates and monitors these sounds, creating noise that moves from loud to soft, from high to low frequency. The test first measures your ability to hear tones of different frequencies, then tests your ability to understand words.

(NEARLY) *I*NVISIBLE HELPERS

If your hearing problems cannot be improved with medical or surgical therapy, you might be a good candidate for a hearing aid. Fortunately, these no longer call to mind that old-fashioned image of a stooped, gnarled, gray-haired woman with a wide plastic device hanging on her ear. Today, hearing aids are compact, miniature, and barely perceptible to others.

Basically, a hearing aid is an amplifier—a miniature version of the one on your stereo. A microphone picks up sound, and the amplifier enhances sound frequencies you wouldn't normally hear. Hearing aids cost anywhere from around $2000—for one so small that before it is inserted into your ear a tiny plastic line must be attached to it so that you can later take it out!—to about $500 for a plastic one that fits on your ear.

The best reason to get a hearing aid? They work! But, remember: They can take some getting used to. Don't be "ampliphobic."

Today's hearing instruments are not the awkward contraptions your grandparents left in the drawer! Give yourself several weeks before deciding that your hearing aid does or doesn't work. And make sure you always have extra batteries in your purse or your car.

Implantable hearing aids will soon be available in the United States, and cochlear implants are already available to those who have a severe-to-profound hearing loss that will not benefit from a hearing aid.

LISTEN TO YOURSELF

Prevention is, as the cliché goes, worth a pound of cure. Although you might not be able to stop aging, you can prevent its early signs from becoming "landmark housing." Ensure the sounds from your back porch are fresh and clear by:

- *Keeping music down* to a level where you don't have to shout to be heard (this goes, if possible, for your teenage son).
- *Being honest.* Tell people you have a hearing problem so they'll talk more slowly and face you when speaking to you.
- *Taking a tip from rock musicians.* Use earplugs if you are in a particularly noisy crowd, movie, or concert.
- *Calling your doctor if you get an ear infection.* Treating the clogged up condition early will help correct the problem more quickly and prevent further complications. Don't wait. Insist on being seen in a timely manner.
- *Cleaning your ears on a regular basis* with a washcloth—and having earwax professionally removed if it builds up.

For more information on hearing loss, contact:

American Tinnitus Association
P. O. Box 5
Portland, OR 97207
1-800-634-8978
(503) 248-9895
(503) 248-0024 (fax)
www.ata.org

Self Help for Hard of Hearing People, Inc.
7910 Woodmont Avenue
Suite 1200
Bethesda, MD 20814
(301) 657-2248
(301) 657-2249 (TTY)
www.shhh.org

Laurent Clerc National Deaf Education Center
Gallaudet University
800 Florida Avenue, NE
Washington, DC 20002
(202) 651-5031 (V/TTY)
www.clercenter.gallaudet.edu

This ends our exploration of your "back porch." It's time now to come back inside—and close the door.

CHAPTER

12

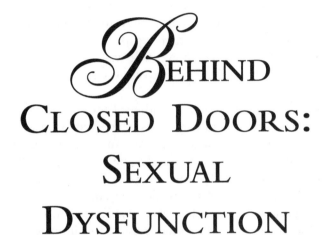

ℬEHIND
CLOSED DOORS:
SEXUAL
DYSFUNCTION

There are always flowers for those who want to see them.
—Henri Matisse

A heart attack would put the fear of God in anyone who survived, at least that's what Anita told herself to explain away the anxiety her husband Paul, a heart attack survivor, seemed to live with. Nor was Paul the only one who was anxious. Anita, too, was terrified it could happen again. They had gotten a second chance, but what if there was a next time? Would they be as lucky?

Paul and Anita's fears went beyond imagining Paul collapsing on the floor of his office, like he did when the first· attack occurred. Theirs was a debilitating fear that it could happen anytime, anywhere—especially during sex.

Anita and Paul had a good, close relationship. They were intimate in the way only couples who have shared a long history can be. They raised two children together; they scrimped and saved and now enjoyed their retirement years in a house by the water. They laughed, they loved, they cried. In short, they lived together, in love, in rhythm.

Except when it came to sex. Of course, in their early twenties, it was hot and heavy. They couldn't wait to get their hands on each other. But, as they got older, as the responsibilities and ups and downs of life prevailed, they found television more of an aphrodisiac than each others' arms.

Sex had become an event. It was still pretty good when they had it, but they didn't have it very often. They were both just too nervous.

The trouble was that neither of them liked the new order of things. There were many times when Anita initiated sex, but Paul rebuffed her out of fear; there were an equal number of times when Paul was "in the mood"—and Anita was the one who said no.

This went on for almost a year. Eventually, neither Anita nor Paul initiated sex; it just made their anxiety worse to be rebuffed or reminded of the horror of Paul's first heart attack. But on another level, both of them missed the intimacy, the loving, in their long relationship. They needed and wanted sex, but it just wasn't happening. They'd begun to bicker; they started not to share as many thoughts and fears and dreams with each other as they had in the past. They had to seek help.

Their family physician suggested they see a therapist. They'd both been suffering from an irrational bout of prolonged anxiety. They were so afraid of Paul having another heart attack that they stayed away from anything the least bit strenuous—and that included sex.

In addition, the hypertensive medications Paul had to take now to control his blood pressure brought his libido down even further. And Anita, her menopausal years behind her, found that her libido was becoming nonexistent.

But this story has a happy ending. After several months in couples therapy, Paul and Anita learned that much of their anxiety had been irrational; it was of their own making. They learned to talk about their problems; they communicated their needs and desires. Paul's doctor also changed his medication to an antihypertensive that wouldn't affect his sex drive; Anita's doctor prescribed a low dose of testosterone to get her libido back in business.

Today, Paul and Anita might not be running around like rabbits whenever they get a chance, but their intimate life is stronger than ever. For a couple in their 70s, they feel very fortunate indeed.

Sex has always been a complicated matter in which physiological issues blend with emotional ones. When we are adolescents and young adults, it is of prime importance to us. Not only are our hormones literally raging through our bodies, but our minds are developing. We're growing and we need to exert our individualities.

As we age, sexuality becomes subdued—or at least sublimated. We learn to accept ourselves as sexual beings, and we are more comfortable with our urges. Physiologically, hormones quiet down, too. We have needs and desires, but we have the ability to keep them in check.

During the "third age" of our lives, sexuality once again goes through an upheaval. Childbearing years are behind us and the onset of menopause creates drops in our sexual hormones, estrogen and testosterone—which, as we have seen with Anita, can affect our drive and our physiology.

Regrettably, the surgical procedures that come with age—hysterectomies, mastectomies, and bypass surgery—can also have a strong impact on sexuality, both emotionally and physically.

Add the libido-decreasing medications that we may need as we age for such conditions as hypertension, diabetes, and depression, and it's no wonder that sexuality as we age has become such a "hot" topic.

But there is good news—a great deal of it, in fact. First of all, because sexuality is so prevalent a theme in the media, we aren't embarrassed to talk about it. There is more communication—which is one of the most important elements in a healthy sex life.

There are also medications available that can help people with sexual dysfunction. We all know about Viagra® and how it has helped millions of men in their middle and senior years; we are learning that Viagra® may help aging women as well. Currently, there is active research on female sexual dysfunction that will eventually yield new medications.

Finally, there are procedures to help men maintain an erection and hormone replacement therapy to help women combat vaginal dryness.

Indeed, there is quite a lot out there to spice up anyone's sexuality—at any age. Let's open the bedroom doors of your house

and examine exactly what causes sexual dysfunction as "your home" ages—and what you can do to stop the problem before it makes its move to your bed.

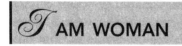 AM WOMAN

Don't worry. This won't be a discussion about the birds and the bees! It also won't be a discussion on the female reproductive cycle. We covered that in *Chapter Six: Hormone Insulation* where we also weighed the pros and cons of hormone replace therapy (HRT) during menopause.

But we will discuss here exactly what menopause mean to a sexually active woman.

In reality: nothing. True, as women age:

- Vaginal dryness can occur.
- The vagina can lose its elasticity and shape.
- More stimulation might be needed in order to reach orgasm.

But other than these few physiological changes, a woman can be sexually active and sexually aroused well into her senior years. In fact, women don't even reach their sexual peak until their 30s.

And that peak has staying power. According to one study, 86% of women in their 40s had sexually active lives, but their number decreased to only 27% after the age of 65. Other studies show that only 20%–40% of 60-year-old women have sex, and that number drops to 15%–30% after the age of 70.

True, a decline in the sexual hormones, estrogen and testosterone, can decrease sexual drive. But the estrogen in HRT can help bring sexual response—being ready and able for sex—right back up. Testosterone supplements, which heighten desire, can help women embrace the joy of sex. And vaginal creams can take care of irritating dryness. So what's the problem?

Part of it is psychological. If a woman, like any human being, thinks she is old, then she will be. If she feels she can no longer be "sexy" after her childbearing years (or if she has had breast surgery or a hysterectomy), then she won't be.

On the other side of this sexual coin, many women find it liberating to be past their childbearing years. It is sexy to them! They

TESTING TESTOSTERONE

DHEA, the new "wonder drug" among natural medicine enthusiasts, has been called a youth serum, an energizer, and a sexual boost. It influences the androgens, or masculine hormones, in your body—in particular, testosterone. DHEA in your body is made in the adrenal gland; testosterone is produced in both the adrenal gland and the ovaries. (DHEA may be dangerous in males and can stimulate both benign and malignant prostate disease. We cannot recommend its use in men.) Check with your doctor since all alternative therapies can have potential side effects.

There are other testosterone supplements available by prescription. If you find that you are lacking in sexual desire, ask your doctor to check your testosterone levels—and, if low, she can prescribe a safe dose of hormone supplement to take.

no longer worry about getting pregnant and can have "pure, unadulterated fun." (Ironically, there's a tribe in Thailand where the senior years of women are celebrated because it does bring a decline in sexual desire—which is seen as a relief!)

But psychology is not enough to explain the decline in sexual activity among senior women. The sad cause, in most cases, is the lack of a partner. Although the statistics are changing, wives still outlive their husbands more often than not. Studies have found that 53% of all women over 65 are widows—and there are only 30 available men for every 100 middle-aged women!

But partner or none, women are learning ways to find sexual satisfaction. They are learning to discard old myths about sexuality and age; they are communicating with their partners and with themselves. Sexual "toys," over-the-counter lubrications such as K-Y Jelly®, and hormone replacement can go far to bring sexual satisfaction to women—and to the men they love as well.

THE BIG E

Estrogen not only balances out your mood, clears your skin, and keeps heart disease at bay. It can also enhance sexual pleasure by keeping the walls of the vagina lubricated and more pliable. It can also reduce vaginal tightness, which can occur when estrogen levels decrease.

*T*HE UNINVITED GUESTS OF SEXUAL DYSFUNCTION: THE 4 "A's"

Some diseases will affect sexual performance in everyone, men and women alike—without you even being aware of why. We call these "gate crashers" the 4 "A's": arthritis, alcohol, anxiety, and antidepressants.

Gate Crasher #1: Arthritis

By its very definition, arthritis can make sexual activity difficult. Perhaps you can't move a certain way, or the pain is so intense you can't think of anything but relief. Ironically, the medications you might take for arthritic pain can make your sexual dysfunction worse. The best solution? Trying out new positions, exercise (under your doctor's supervision), or a change of medication. The good news—the endorphins released during orgasm have been shown to increase the performance of arthritics in other activities.

Gate Crasher #2: Alcohol Abuse

Alcohol has always been seen as an aphrodisiac, a drug that releases inhibitions and fuels desire. In reality, alcohol has the opposite effect. Drink too much and all you'll wind up doing in bed is sleeping it off. Alcohol is a direct depressant of sexual function, potentially causing impotency in men and reducing the inability to have an orgasm in women.

Gate Crasher #3: Anxiety

Paul and Anita, our examples in the beginning of this chapter, are not alone. Many men who suffer a heart attack are terrified that they'll have another one—during sex. And many women who love them are equally scared it will happen again—during sex. This fear becomes a part of a vicious cycle: the disease, which can create impotency, and the fear of disease, which may make the disease worse!

It is time to put these fears to rest. Studies show that there is virtually no proof that sexual activity can precipitate a heart attack. In fact, only 1% of all coronary-based sudden deaths occur during sex. The amount of energy and oxygen the sexual act uses is minimum—the equivalent of walking up the stairs. Cardiologists usually suggest waiting only 12 to 16 weeks after a heart attack to have sex.

So if your doctor gives you the green light, go for it! (But take off your Nikes® first!)

Gate Crasher #4: Antidepressants

For some reason, the very medications that decrease depression by increasing the levels of serotonin in your brain can also decrease the chemicals that excite the libido. These antidepressants, called the SSRI's, include Prozac®, Effexor®, Paxil®, and Zoloft®. Fortunately, medications can be changed, and there are enough antidepressants available for your physician to find one that relieves your depression without sexual side-effects.

A diminished sexual drive does not have to be your fate as you age. In fact the media are filled with stories of people meeting and falling in love in their 60s, 70s, and even their 80s! And many married couples enjoy a healthy sex life well into their senior years.

As we have seen throughout the pages of this book, life does not end with middle age. It doesn't end with old age. Yes, things change, things are different. But *Vive la différence!*

Here's some ways to keep your "drive alive":

Drive Alive #1: Talk to Each Other

Good communications is the key to success: in business, in the community, in life. It is also crucial in sexual relationships. You need to be able to express your frustrations and your fears. There's also the power of two: You might discover solutions you couldn't see on your own. Don't be shy. Don't be embarrassed. Talk about how you feel. Discuss what would enhance your pleasure. Be honest. And, while you're making time for talk, make time for intimacy, too!

Drive Alive #2: Schedule Sex

Sure, you might lose some spontaneity, but scheduling intimacy is important in your busy life. Just as there are many freedoms as you age, there are stresses, too. The children being out of the house can buy you personal space, but it can also make you feel lonely. Retirement will give you the chance to try all the things you have not yet done, but adjusting to your new routine can be overwhelming. Health, too, can be an issue as you age; you tire more quickly. All the more reason to schedule time together—before you take a nap.

Drive Alive #3: Create Your Own Definition of Sex

Sex is not a Victoria's Secret ad. Nor is it a *Gone with the Wind* moment. Sex can mean many different things to people. Intimacy, closeness, sharing of thoughts and touch, these can go far in making you feel good—without the sexual act itself. If you don't feel the pressure to perform, you just might outperform yourself later!

Drive Alive #4: Be Assertive

One of the main reasons older people don't have frequent sex is that they lack partners. Widowhood, divorce, illness—these take their toll and you can be left flying solo. But you don't have to spend your nights in front of the TV.

Get out there. Take a class. Join a club. Let your friends know you are interested in meeting someone. Check out Web sites and personal ads (but never give out your real name and address, at least initially). Be proactive. You'll never know when you might meet a special someone—who is also looking for you.

Drive Alive #5: Take Care of Yourself

The best aphrodisiac? Health. There's nothing like the glow of well-being to put a spring in your step, a sheen to your skin, a smile on your face. Get the glow with a healthy, low-fat diet; regular exercise; and a solid night's sleep. Get physical check-ups regularly to ensure your continued health—and to take care of any problems early on. Talk to your doctor if you have any concerns— from sex to nutrition, from fatigue to aches and pains. She's there to help.

For more information on sexual dysfunction, contact:

National Council on Aging
409 3rd Street SW, Suite 200
Washington, DC 20024
(800) 424-9046
(202) 479-0735
www.ncoa.org

National Institute on Aging
NIA Information Center
Box 8057
Gaithersburg, MD 20898
(800) 222-2225
(800) 222-4225 (TTY)
www.nih.gov/nia/health

Sexual Function Health Council
1128 North Charles Street
Baltimore, MD 21201
(410) 468-1800
www.afud.org

We've now opened the bedroom doors on sexual dysfunction. Let's move on to your private chambers: bladder and bowel dysfunction.

CHAPTER

13

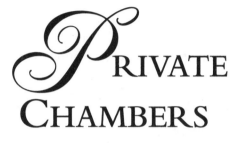

PRIVATE CHAMBERS

Knowledge comes, but wisdom lingers.
—Alfred, Lord Tennyson

At first, it was only a few drops when she laughed—and Rosemary laughed quite a bit. She even giggled about it with her friends; they all said it was a sign of age. "Don't cough," they'd say over lunch. "Don't sneeze. Don't laugh. And wear panty shields at all times!"

Rosemary went on laughing—until the morning she woke up and discovered that she had wet herself in the middle of the night.

Rosemary was mortified, horrified. She made a silent prayer of thanks that she lived alone. She quickly got out of bed, bathed herself and threw the bedding in the wash. She was a little scared but she chose to ignore it. How could she tell someone what had happened? After all, she was 62 years old, not a toddler!

Rosemary had had a mild stroke two years before but her neurologist had been very pleased with her progress. She'd been left with a slight paralysis on her right side—that was all; she couldn't open jars or carry heavy items with her right hand as well as she could before. And she never had a problem with incontinence! That hadn't even come up after her stroke.

So what was wrong?

Unfortunately, Rosemary continued to ignore her problem. She went to a drugstore on the other side of town and purchased a box of disposable panties. She didn't tell any of her friends what was going on when they next had lunch; she wore a skirt so they wouldn't see the bulge of what she called her "secret diapers."

But, as often proves true, eventually the things you ignore resurface—and you cannot deny them anymore. For Rosemary the situation changed when an angry rash developed on her inner thigh and she felt a burning sensation every time she urinated.

It was time to seek help.

Rosemary is not alone—in either her incontinence or her "shame." Approximately 10 million Americans have the same problem—and many of them did not see a doctor until the pain and discomfort grew too difficult to ignore. That's unfortunate. Because more than 70% of all cases of incontinence can be cured—or at least treated successfully.

Rosemary finally got the help she needed. It turned out that her leakage had so irritated her bladder and her thighs that she had developed a severe urinary tract infection. Left untreated, it might have affected her kidneys.

The doctor diagnosed Rosemary's condition as urge incontinence; she had lost some of her control over voiding. Most likely, it had been a residual symptom of her stroke, worsened by the weakening of the bladder muscles brought on by age. She was given specific pelvic exercises called Kegel exercises plus biofeedback to strengthen the muscles that supported her bladder, pelvis, and uterus. She was also given an antibiotic that would get rid of her urinary infection.

Today, armed with knowledge, a support group of other incontinent people, and her Kegel exercises, Rosemary leads a completely full and normal life.

Even better, she's no longer concerned about wetting herself when she laughs. That should be the worst of her problems!

We don't talk a lot about elimination, either by the bladder or the bowel. And yet, it is a crucial process for our body; outside of sweating from our pores, it is the only way we can get rid of waste and toxins.

So what's the problem? Why do we keep the bladder and the bowel in the private chambers of our house? Why do we ignore problems that are so easily treatable—and that can be quite dangerous if ignored?

It's time now for this "old house" to open the windows (in the bathroom and in every room!) and let the sun pour in—starting with the not-so-private urinary tract.

⒯HE URINARY TRACT

It's not something we think about it—until we have to go. The need to urinate is almost a reflex; when we feel the urge nothing will relieve it except to go. Whether driving in the car with no restroom in sight, sitting at your grandchild's piano recital, or watching the last inning of the World Series, when you have to go, you have to go. Just like that, in seconds, the need that is practically a reflex—basic and not part of your consciousness—becomes the only thing you can think about. You can "hold it in" seemingly forever, but the need becomes a driving force in your brain, stronger than making time in the car, listening to your grandchild play the piano, or finding out who wins the World Series.

But what if that urge were uncontrollable? Or if you didn't feel the urge to go? Or if accidents happened that you couldn't stop? Suddenly, elimination would become a very important aspect of your life.

These problems do occur—in three-quarters of our population, especially in the "golden years." Fortunately, solutions are plentiful—as long as you communicate your problems to your doctor. But first things first. In order to understand the conditions that can arise within the urinary tract, you need to know where they can happen and why. You need a "blueprint" of this particular room.

Whether it's a piece of fruit or a charcoal-grilled steak, eventually all the food we eat is broken down into liquids. By the time food (now liquid) reaches our small intestines, it is further broken down into the most minute chemical components. Nutrients are absorbed by the body and utilized as cell food. Waste, on the other hand, is sent to the kidneys through the bloodstream. (We'll be discussing solid waste later on in this chapter—which, instead of

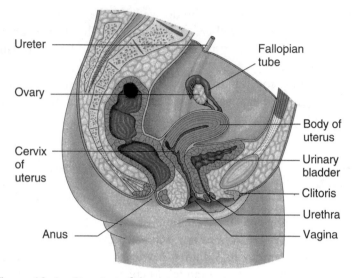

Figure 13–1 Drawing of the urinary tract in a woman

going to the kidneys, goes to the large intestines for elimination.) Basically, the kidneys act as filters, "cleaning" the blood and separating it even further, into life-sustaining fluids, which are sent back into the bloodstream as waste, which needs to be eliminated. This waste travels down thin tubes called ureters, one on either side of the kidneys, to the bladder, where it is held until the "urge" to "go" passes it out through the urethra. (In men, the urethra is also a receptacle for sperm.)

The pelvic muscles help keep waste where it belongs, in the bladder, until you're ready to relieve yourself. How do you know when to go? Enter the nervous system, which helps you determine when you can go—and when you have to hold it in. When the bladder gets full, a messenger is dispatched via the spinal cord to the brain to say, "I'm uncomfortable."

The brain, in turn, tells your legs to get moving and find a bathroom fast. It also sends a message to the base of the spinal cord, where a group of nerves called the reflex arc initiate the actual voiding reflex when "the coast is clear." Bladder muscles then contract, pushing urine into the urethra and out the body.

That's it. Different systems working together. Clear-cut and incredibly efficient—until something goes wrong.

𝓑LADDER BLATHER

Although incontinence can occur at any age, it is most prevalent in "seniors" whose muscles grow weaker as they grow older. Women have even more of a problem because their pelvic floor—the tissues and muscles that help support the reproductive system—begins to sag after childbirth. The drop in estrogen levels during menopause also causes the walls of the urinary tract to thin—which can further weaken the pelvic muscles. The result? Leakage when you least expect it.

Incontinence is just a fancy word for this involuntary release of urine. The condition is common and it's treatable—if you speak up, as Rosemary eventually did, and talk to your doctor about your situation.

There is incontinence, however, and then there is more incontinence. In fact, there are three distinct types; many people experience more than one. To help you understand the variables of incontinence, let's go over the three "Wet Ones."

Wet One #1: Stress Incontinence

This is the least obtrusive of the three—and the most common. In stress incontinence, the muscles around the urethra that keep waste in the bladder where it belongs, are weakened. Any sudden pressure on the bladder, a cough, a sneeze, a laugh, even exercising, can "open the floodgates"—although usually only a few drops worth. Leakage is negligible and problems can be kept in check with Kegel exercises plus biofeedback, panty liners, and personal hygiene.

Wet Ones #2: Urge Incontinence

This one goes to the "brain" of the matter. Your brain never receives the message that your bladder is full, and you have no control over the need to "let loose."

In urge incontinence, you are like a toddler, unable to hold your urine. Understandably, this "wet one" is one of the more difficult to accept; it affects our basic needs and early training.

DO THE KEGEL

No, it's not a kind of ethnic pastry. It's not a new interior designer from Europe. Kegel is a series of exercises developed to strengthen the muscles in the pelvic floor that support and control contractions in the reproductive organs, in the bladder, and the urethra. The exercises remind the brain to pay attention "down there".

The Kegel exercises themselves are a study in control. While you are urinating, slowly "push in" or contract your pelvis. This stops the flow of urine. Hold for 10 seconds, then release. Repeat five or six times.

You can also do Kegel at other times—at the gym, while you're sitting and watching television, while you're still in bed, while you're brushing your teeth, or even while standing on line at the bank. The more you Kegel, the more you'll be able to control your elimination.

Urge incontinence usually occurs in people who have had a stroke or who have developed neurological disorders such as multiple sclerosis, Alzheimer's disease, and Parkinson's disease. It is also one of the early signs of bladder cancer. But urge incontinence can also have a less serious root; it can be a function of decreased estrogen levels and simply a "normal" part of aging.

Wet One #3: Overflow Incontinence

Here, the bladder is never quite emptied. The "release and void" signals from the brain go unheard and, consequently, you never quite eliminate enough. Urine "pools" in the bladder; spillover leakage occurs. This "wet one" can occur in women who have diabetes, fibroids, or an ovarian tumor.

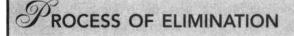ROCESS OF ELIMINATION

If you think you have leakage problems, the first step is to see your doctor or a urologist (a specialist in the urinary tract). The doctor will take a complete medical history and perform a physical exam to make sure you have no tumors. If necessary, he will also perform a:

- *Urine test.* This is the reason for the "little cup" when you go to the doctor's office. This test is the first step in determining if you have diabetes or a urinary tract infection (UTI).
- *Urine culture.* If your physician thinks a UTI may be present, he'll send a urine specimen to the lab. Here, several drops of urine will be placed in a culture medium; if any bacteria—and what type—is present in your urine, it will grow. If you have a UTI, the results from the culture will help determine which antibiotic would be most effective against it.
- *Uroflowmeter.* In this test you must drink fluids and fill up your bladder. You'll then urinate into a machine which determines the amount, intensity, and speed at which your urine flows.
- *Cystometry.* In more stubborn cases a urologist might insert thin, snake-like tubes—similar to those used in a colonoscopy to check your lower intestinal tract—into your bladder to determine the strength of your pelvic muscles and bladder by seeing how much pressure they can exert during contractions.

ℒIFE AFTER INCONTINENCE

Although not life-threatening, incontinence can hamper your lifestyle. It can also create emotional problems, making you feel "old" before your time.

It doesn't have to be that way. There are many techniques, products, medications, and treatments available to help. Some of these include:

- *Bladder retraining.* In addition to doing Kegel exercises, refashioning your mind to follow an elimination pattern can go far to prevent accidents. For one week, you'll be asked to keep a "urine diary," recording the times you go to the bathroom, as well as the amounts and types of fluids you drink. You'll also make scheduled "bathroom trips" every half-hour or hour. Eventually, you will become aware of when you need to void. By regulating the amount of fluids you drink and by going to the bathroom at specific times each day, you help your body "learn" to eliminate at the appropriate time. (*Retraining also works with constipation and other stool problems. See the section on the bowel later in this chapter.*)

- *Medications* such as Flomax®, Detrol®, and Ditropan®, can help stop your incontinence by controlling the muscles that contract and open during urination. (Side effects may include dry mouth and eye problems.) If you are in menopause, your doctor may also prescribe hormone replacement therapy (*see Chapter Six*) to help strengthen your urinary tract walls. Your doctor will also prescribe an antibiotic for any UTI your incontinence may have caused.

- *Pessaries* are devices for women that help control incontinence. They are inserted into the vagina to support the pelvic floor.

- *Vaginal weights* are the equivalent of hand-held weights—but designed for your pelvis. These small, cone-shaped weights, in varying degrees of heaviness, are inserted into your vagina as you perform Kegel-like exercises. Eventually, your pelvic wall becomes stronger and you are more able to control your incontinence.

- *Biofeedback* techniques help control incontinence in approximately 50% of patients. A catheter is inserted into the urethra and fluid is "pumped" into the bladder. At the same time, you resist the urge to urinate with biofeedback (a training tool which helps you become aware of changes in body temperature and function when you need to go). Ultimately, you "teach" your body to wait.

- *Injectable agents* such as the collagen used by plastic surgeons to plump up wrinkles can now be injected directly into a woman's urinary sphincter. The collagen enlarges the sphincter, improving control.

- *Valvular devices* can be inserted directly into a woman's urethra. When a woman performs a valsalva maneuver (similar to bearing down to have a bowel movement), the valve opens 8–10 seconds later and remains open for three minutes. The valve remains in place for several months and is then replaced. These devices are currently in the final phases of study and they should be released soon.

- *Surgery* can repair weak pelvic walls when all else fails. Surgeons can also help reduce blockage and reposition the bladder. A catheter can also be inserted into the urethra to collect urine that is then deposited into a container. (If you find you need a catheter, it is crucial to be clean. Personal hygiene is vital to avoid infection.)

CRANBERRIES ARE NOT JUST FOR THANKSGIVING

Studies have found that drinking cranberry juice every day can prevent urinary tract infections. The juice makes the walls of the bladder and urethra too "slippery" for bacteria to cling to and grow. If you're afraid of the sugar and the calories, simply swallow two cranberry capsules a day. You can find them in your health food store.

For more information on incontinence, contact:

National Association for Continence
P.O. Box 8306
Spartanburg, SC 29305
(800) BLADDER
www.nafc.org

The Simon Foundation
P.O. Box 835-F
Willamette, IL 60091
(800) 23-SIMON
www.simonfoundation.org

ℐDJOINING ROOMS: THE REST OF THE STORY

As the commercials tell us, irregularity is no picnic. Constipation can make you feel tired, cranky, bloated, and gassy. It is not pleasant, but join the club. Almost everyone, at some time in their lives, has been constipated. You take a laxative, a stool softener, or an antacid and the symptoms disappear.

But what if constipation becomes, well, constant? If, as you age, it becomes an uncomfortable fact of life?

When you digest food (*see Chapter Fifteen for an in-depth look at the gastrointestinal tract*), not all of it is broken down and absorbed by the body. Some of the food by-product you eat is solid waste—which, like urine, must be eliminated. Solid waste

is stored in the large intestine, becoming bulkier and bulkier with the fiber you eat, additional waste, and other by-products until you feel the urge to eliminate—and the waste passes out the rectum and the anus as stool.

As with urination, a bowel movement is not something you give much thought to—until you have to go. That need to "go" differs with every person. Some people have regular bowel movements—that only occur twice a week. Still others have a regular bowel movement twice a day. The "once a day" adage is really a myth; everyone is different, with a different body, and if you are comfortable, you don't have a problem—no matter how little or how much you go.

Constipation becomes an issue, however, if you have:

- difficulty passing stools
- pain
- blood in your stools
- bloating
- the need to go without the ability to do so

If you have any of these symptoms, you need to see your doctor to make sure you aren't showing signs of a more serious condition. (*See Chapter Fifteen for some of the diseases that can affect the gastrointestinal tract in your senior years.*) Constipation itself is not serious as much as it is uncomfortable. Some of the reasons behind "stubborn stool" include:

Stubborn Stool #1: Lack of Fiber

One of the reasons constipation is so common in the elderly is because of dietary change. Older people tend to eat fewer fresh fruits and vegetables—that provide the bulk and fiber needed for regularity. As an older person, you might lose interest in cooking—or not be able to cook up a storm like you used to. Or you might find that fiber-rich food gives you gas and makes you feel bloated. Thus, instead of steamed asparagus, you might opt for mashed potatoes. Instead of salad, you'll opt for butter-cooked stringbeans.

Stubborn Stool #2: Medication

It's a fact of life: Older people take more medicine. One of the side-effects of this medicine can be constipation. Diuretics, antidepressants, antihistamines, high blood pressure medication, even antiacids, can cause irregularity.

Stubborn Stool #3: Not Enough Fluids

Many of us don't drink enough water. The American Dietetic Association recommends drinking six to eight glasses of water a day, but many of us don't even get close. And caffeniated beverages, such as soda, coffee, and tea, "soak up" whatever liquids we do consume. Dehydration is not uncommon in older people. And that dehydration can cause constipation, too.

Stubborn Stool #4: Disease

It's easy to see where bowel-specific diseases can cause irregularity. Colorectal cancer, irritable bowel syndrome, diverticulitis—these can all create constipation. But did you know that multiple sclerosis, depression, Parkinson's disease, and diabetes can also cause constipation? Another good reason to get yourself to the doctor if you experience irregularity!

Stubborn Stool #5: Laxative Misuse

Maybe as a teenager, it seems "cool" to take a laxative and lose unwanted pounds with your dinner. This debilitating behavior can follow some people their whole lives—until they become so dependent on laxatives they can't go to the bathroom without them. Or perhaps you bought an over-the-counter laxative for a bout of constipation and took it a little longer than recommended. When this occurs, your body can actually "forget" how to have a bowel movement without an artificial prompt. The best bet is to do things naturally: A stool softener can help, as can psyllium seeds.

Stubborn Stool #6: Lack of Exercise

Exercise is crucial for regularity. If you are a sedentary person, your elimination system is not going to work efficiently. If you take a walk every day—getting that blood pumped, those arms and legs moving—you'll not only be helping your cardiovascular system, you'll be aiding digestion and elimination, too. Your body won't have to work as hard to do its job.

BULK ORDERS

One of the most effective ways to treat constipation is with fiber. Eat a diet rich in fresh fruits and vegetables, peanut butter, lentils and other legumes, and whole grains. If your stomach cannot handle fiber-rich food, make sure you take a psyllium seed product mixed with water or juice every day. Metamucil®, for example, is widely available in drugstores.

Stubborn Stool #7: Self-Consciousness

Some people are embarrassed by the natural process of elimination. The phenomenon is so common that an episode of Seinfeld focused on George not being able to go to the bathroom while on a date with a new girlfriend. The problem with this kind of self-conscious behavior is that once the urge has passed, it might not come again for a while.

For more information on constipation, contact the:

**National Digestive Diseases Information
Clearinghouse**
Box NDDIC
Bethesda, MD 20892
(301) 654-3810
(301) 907-8906 (fax)
www.niddk.nih.gov/health/digest/nddic.htm

Digestive Disease National Coalition
711 Second Street NE, Suite 200
Washington, DC 20002
(202) 544-7497
(202) 546-7105 (fax)
www.ddnc.org

It's time now to leave the upper floors of your house and check out the heating units—specifically the circulation, lungs, and heart conditions that can occur as you age.

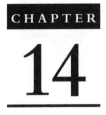

CHAPTER

14

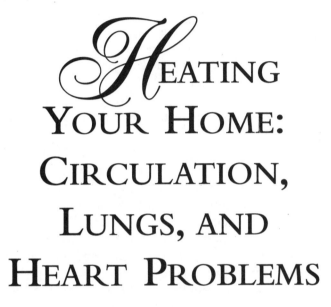

HEATING YOUR HOME: CIRCULATION, LUNGS, AND HEART PROBLEMS

There is only one way to happiness and that is to cease worrying about things which are beyond the power of our will.
—Epictetus

It was sudden, quiet. Janet never saw it coming. But one moment she was taking her dog for a walk in the beautiful sunshine, the next she was doubled over in pain.

Janet began to sweat; she felt a sharp pain on her left side; she gasped. Her dog howling and leaping around her, Janet sagged down to the curb. She thought she had had a terrible gas pain and she rued the fried chicken meal she had had the night before.

Slowly, in a few moments, Janet's breath came back. The sweat cooled on her brow. She patted her dog's head, slowly got back up, and limped home.

Her husband was in the kitchen getting ready to go to work. He took one look at Janet and almost dropped his coffee. She looked pale, waxy. Worse, she looked worried. He made her sit down and tell him what happened.

Five minutes later, they were on their way to the hospital. Janet kept saying she didn't need to go; she was fine. Her husband ignored her. She most definitely wasn't fine.

The emergency room doctor didn't need to be a cardiologist to know what had happened to Janet. She'd had a mild heart attack. "You were lucky," he said.

Janet didn't consider herself very lucky, but the doctor persisted. "You can change things. You can stop the disease from progressing."

The attack had been a warning, a clanging bell that intoned for Janet to shape up—or literally ship out.

But where to start? Janet felt overwhelmed, scared. So did her husband. Janet's doctor reassured her at her next visit. Janet's fears were very common in people who have had a heart attack. Fear of death, worry about every little stab of pain, depression, a feeling of being out of control—all these and more are very real to a person with a heart condition.

The most successful solution, however, was within Janet's control. She had to change her life: start a low-fat diet, begin an exercise routine, practice stress-reducing strategies, and take one aspirin every day. Simple, easy—and it could help prevent another attack from taking place.

Janet's story is more typical than you might think. Millions of people past the age of 40 worry about heart disease. And with good reason: 95% of all heart attacks occur in people who are middle-aged. Heart disease is the cause of 40% of all deaths in people between the ages of 65 and 74. It is also one of the major causes of disability in old age.

Even more sobering: Heart disease is the number one cause of death in women in America—and yet most of us either choose to ignore its symptoms or worry far more about cancer. We just don't think it will happen to us. According to the American Heart Association, only 10% of all American women realize the devastation heart disease can wrought. In fact, women are ten times more likely to die of a heart attack than breast cancer.

Heart disease is becoming such a concern in women over 65, in fact, that the National Cholesterol Education Program of the National Heart, Lung, and Blood Institute recommended substantial changes in the number of people who should take cholesterol-reducing drugs—from 13 million to 36 million Americans! They recommend that even women on HRT should not rely on the increased estrogen to protect them if they have high cholesterol, diabetes, hypertension, or a poor lifestyle.

Another problem is that most women don't realize what a heart attack entails. It is not always a crushing pain followed by oblivion. Heart attacks in women do not always cause chest pain. Instead, they may become dizzy or light-headed; they might feel pain in their jaws, arms, or bellies instead of in the chest. Even more ironic: most chest pains in women are not caused by a heart attack.

Studies bear this out. A 1999 study found that women who had heart attacks delayed going to the hospital. To make matters worse, when they did get to the emergency room, they weren't given the proper emergency medicines: aspirin and other blood thinners and beta-blocker medications.

Yet it is crucial for women to understand the ramifications of heart disease: Women don't fare as well with bypass surgery. They are also more likely to die after a heart attack or have a second one six years after the first.

Why are women so susceptible to heart disease? The answer might lie in a woman's predilection to "take on the world"—and everyone in it. Women are pulled in many more directions than men: Family, career, and friends. On the whole, they worry more. Coupled with their denial that they will not have a heart attack and the risk climbs.

What makes all this so worrisome is the fact that heart disease can, for the most part, be prevented by making healthier lifestyle choices.

It simply doesn't have to be a killer. True, someone who is 75 years old will have a greater risk of developing heart disease; the "ticker" is older, more worn. But, the risk can be lowered if (and it's an important if) a woman becomes more aware of her heart— and if she eats right, exercises, doesn't smoke, and tries to keep calm.

Heart disease, circulatory problems, and respiratory conditions are all real-life scenarios for aging baby boomers. But they can be controlled; they can be kept at bay. In the same way that maintaining the heating system in your home will keep you warm and

toasty in winter, keeping your heart and lungs healthy will help ensure a long, energetic life.

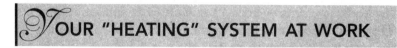

YOUR "HEATING" SYSTEM AT WORK

Before you can understand how things can go wrong, you have to recognize how they work "right." To that end, here is a brief education into the way your home is heated—via your heart, lungs, and circulatory system.

Like the brain, which is so small and so powerful, the heart—which is no bigger than a fist—is absolutely crucial for life.

The heart is a muscle, an efficient, never-ceasing pump, which is the center of a dynamic circle. The circle begins as oxygen-rich blood—the food our body eats—is pumped from the lungs and sent throughout the body in blood vessels called arteries. Once our cells have "eaten" their fill of oxygen, the now- depleted blood travels back to the heart in vessels called veins. Back at the heart, the oxygen-depleted blood is then pumped back up to the lungs to pick up more food.

Of course, the circulatory system is much more complicated than this. There are interconnecting vessels and passageways and tunnels—all whose express purpose is bringing oxygen and nutrients to hungry cells. The heart itself is divided into four nearly symmetrical chambers; entry and exit are governed by valves that open and close as blood is pushed and pumped. When the heart muscle relaxes, oxygen-rich blood from the lungs rushes through

- The *pulmonary veins* into
- The *left atrium,* which sends it past the mitral valve into the
- *Left ventricle.* When the heart muscle contracts, the motion pumps and pushes the oxygen-rich blood up and out past the aortic valve to the
- *Aorta,* the largest artery in the body, which branches out into a complex network of smaller arteries. This network carries oxygen to the cells in every part of your body as the heart continues to relax and contract, push and pump, relax and contract.
- After the cells have eaten, the now oxygen-depleted blood (which also contains carbon dioxide waste) travels back to the heart via a network of veins which leads to the *superior and inferior vena cava*

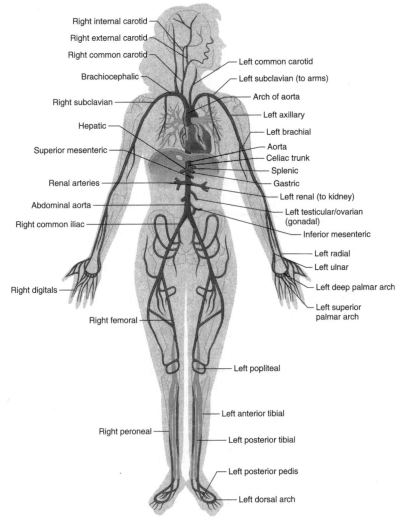

Figure 14–1 Drawing of a heart and its arteries.

- which lead up to and end in the *right atrium*
- The oxygen-depleted blood then travels past the *tricuspid valve* down to the *right ventricle*, where it is pumped up and out to the lungs to get more "food."

The heart is the major element in our circulatory system, which consists of all those arteries and veins and capillaries (tiny blood vessels) that send and retrieve blood throughout our bodies. Problems can arise in many places throughout the system: within the chambers of the heart; at the valves, where blood is

rhythmically pumped and pushed into different chambers and out into the body, or within the blood vessels themselves.

$\mathcal{L}$UNG LORE

The lungs, although technically a part of the respiratory system, are a crucial component of heart health. It is through the air we breathe that oxygen is gathered—and through which waste, in the form of carbon dioxide, is expelled.

When we breathe in air through our nose and mouth, the air travels down into our lungs through the trachea (also called the windpipe), then through airways, or tubes, which branch out deep within our lungs.

The larger of these branching tubes are called bronchi; the smaller tubes, imbedded deep within lung tissue, are called bronchioles. Deeper still are minute airway sacs called alveoli. It is here, within the alveoli, that oxygen-rich air mingles with the carbon monoxide-rich blood from the heart. Oxygen is passed to the blood; carbon monoxide is passed from the blood into the alveoli. This process is called diffusion—and it is the basis of all life.

The oxygen-rich blood then travels to the heart; the "waste-filled" air travels out of the lungs and is expelled when we exhale.

As we age, problems can occur in the lungs because they can scar, decrease in volume, and decrease their ability to exchange oxygen and carbon monoxide. If the blood going through the lungs doesn't pick up enough oxygen, our heart doesn't get enough to pass along to all our cells.

In short, the lungs, the heart, and the circulatory systems are all connected—so a problem in one will affect the whole process.

$\mathcal{H}$EART MURMURS: PROBLEMS OF THE HEART

Despite everything we know today about heart health, cardiovascular disease is still the number one killer among American men over 40 and American women over 60 (when estrogen levels decline).

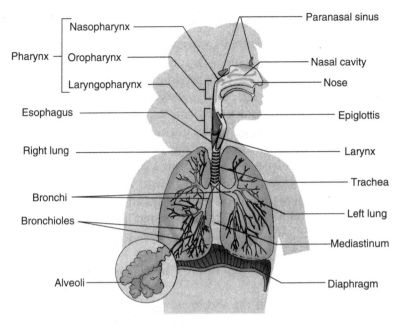

Figure 14–2 Drawing of the lungs

The physical causes of heart disease have less to do with the aging heart—healthy heart muscle does not grow weaker—than with the aging of the body in general: Lung capacity declines; artery walls grow thicker (in a process called atherosclerosis); and maximum heart rate declines.

Normal aging is not the problem. Natural aging—and even some hardening of the arteries—doesn't interfere with a long and healthy life. Indeed, there are marathon runners going the distance well into their 70s. There are yoga experts, personal trainers, and physical education teachers who never dream of retiring.

But sometimes heredity or poor living habits (or a combination of the two) interfere with the heart's ability to get enough oxygen or maintain blood flow to do its jobs. Valves leading from one chamber to the next can malfunction, stick or leak over time. Atherosclerosis can become so severe that it blocks the flow of blood from the heart. It can also block the blood supply that feeds the heart muscle itself. This is when heart disease can set in.

Some of the more common "heart darts" that can occur in aging baby boomers include:

Heart Dart #1: Atherosclerosis

The most common cause of a myocardial infarction—the official name for a heart attack—is a hardening, or thickening, of the arteries to the point where they become blocked and oxygen-rich blood cannot get through. This narrowing of the arteries leading to the heart is a condition called coronary heart disease.

Here's how it happens: In the normal wear and tear of living, fatty deposits grow in streaks on the inside of artery walls; over time, these walls can erode and become damaged. As new tissue eventually grows over the damaged areas, scars and tiny bumps may develop. Over time, these tiny bumps attract cholesterol, fatty deposits, and white blood cells—creating plaque. This plaque builds up and eventually blocks the arteries, preventing blood and oxygen from flowing normally. If the plaque breaks open or splits, it clogs the artery and can cause a heart attack, or myocardial infarction.

The large artery in the abdomen, the aorta, can also "balloon out" and form an aneurysm that can rupture. Early identification can lead to life-saving surgical repair. (*See the information on surgery later in this chapter.*)

Atherosclerosis may be a normal part of aging, but it doesn't have to be a debilitating one. Not every aging baby boomer develops heart disease. Some of the risk factors are:

- *High levels of cholesterol,* particularly LDL, or "bad" cholesterol, which clings to artery walls. LDL cholesterol is a double whammy. Not only does it promote plaque, it also combines with free radical molecules (pesky toxins from certain foods, preservatives, and the environment that antioxidants love to "eat") to hinder transport of cholesterol through the arteries, creating even more damage to arterial walls. (*Cholesterol-lowering drugs can substantially reduce a woman's risk of heart disease. See preventative measures later in this chapter.*)

- *High blood pressure,* or hypertension. Called the "silent disease," high blood pressure can be a killer if it's not treated. In order for your body to get the oxygen-rich "food" it needs, blood must be pumped with considerable pressure to push it through your arteries. Your blood pressure is the amount of this pressure exerted against artery walls. As age stiffens arteries and makes them less elastic, more pressure is needed to get that blood moving. The more pressure your heart must use to get past stiff artery walls, the more the chance of plaque build

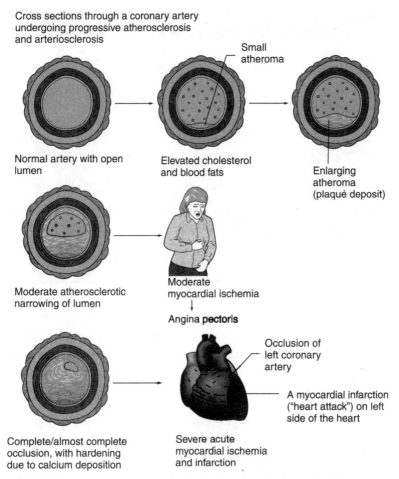

Cross sections through a coronary artery undergoing progressive atherosclerosis and arteriosclerosis

Small atheroma

Normal artery with open lumen

Elevated cholesterol and blood fats

Enlarging atheroma (plaque deposit)

Moderate atherosclerotic narrowing of lumen

Moderate myocardial ischemia

↓

Angina **pectoris**

Occlusion of left coronary artery

A myocardial infarction ("heart attack") on left side of the heart

Complete/almost complete occlusion, with hardening due to calcium deposition

Severe acute myocardial ischemia and infarction

Figure 14–3 The build-up of atherosclerosis which can lead to a heart attack.

up and damage. It becomes a vicious cycle: the more plaque, the more damage to artery walls—and the more pressure the heart has to exert. Eventually, artery walls get so blocked with plaque that blood cannot get through. Worse, the heart itself gets overworked and can become damaged. (*High blood pressure medication can keep hypertension under control. See preventative measures later in this chapter.*)

- *Cigarette smoking.* If it isn't obvious yet how damaging cigarette smoking can be, here's more proof: Carbon monoxide, found in cigarettes, damages arterial walls and can cause heart disease.
- *Stress.* It's easy to see how stress—the unrelenting kind—can create more tension on your heart, forcing it to beat faster and

A NEW URINE TEST

You can now urinate in a cup to determine whether you are at risk for heart disease. According to *Circulation*, the journal of the American Heart Association, the protein albumen may be linked to heart disease. A study of over 1,100 post-menopausal women in the Netherlands found that 4.4 times as many women who died from heart disease had high levels of albumen in their urine—as opposed to women who had no traces of the protein in their urine. A simple, routine urine test in your doctor's office can see if you have increased levels of albumen in your body—and if you are at risk.

harder. But creating plaque buildup? Atherosclerosis? Yes. In fact, in one particular study, people living in a war-zone country had much greater plaque build up than their counterparts who lived in more peaceful areas. It is not stress in general, but the "hostility" factor of a Type A personality that correlates with heart disease.

- *Obesity.* If you are overweight, the chances are good that you are on your way of developing atherosclerolic damage; excess weight puts strain on your heart and arteries. Obesity is also linked to a high-fat diet—which is linked to high cholesterol and diabetes.

- *Sedentary lifestyle.* Exercise has been found to increase HDL, or "good" cholesterol, in the body. HDL works like a vacuum cleaner, gobbling up LDL deposits clinging to artery walls and helping to make the flow of arterial blood more efficient. If you are a couch potato, chances are you're not only suffering from lack of exercise but eating poorly—and overweight—to boot.

Heart Dart #2: Angina

Think of a sudden, new and unusual, sensation in your chest and you'll have an idea what angina feels like. Angina is more of an ache than a pain—an ache like heartburn or a cramp. Angina's ability to masquerade as something else (e.g., heartburn or gas)

WHO'S CLAUDE?

If you are experiencing leg cramps or an aching sensation in our thighs or calves when you are working hard, they might not be simple muscle strain. If the pains go away after a few minutes of rest, you could have an angina-like ache called intermittent claudication. In normal language, this means that your arteries in your pelvis, thighs, or calves are blocked as a result of atherosclerosis. The best way to know? Make an appointment to see your doctor as soon as you can.

leads to the fact that it is often ignored. The result of coronary heart disease (in particular atherosclerosis of the coronary arteries), angina occurs when the heart is overworked and not getting enough oxygen.

If you get angina pangs during a bout of strenuous exercise, after a heavy meal, or after exposure to cold, your angina is considered stable and it is usually temporary. Think of it as a *warning sign* of heart disease, a signal that the heart, for a moment, was momentarily stimulated—either through exertion, digestion, or change in temperature—to work harder. But angina that comes on while you are watching TV or, in Janet's case in our opening example, walking the dog, can be a sign of a more serious heart condition. (To be safe, seek immediate attention if you suffer any angina-like pangs.)

Left untreated, angina can cause myocardial infarction and even sudden death. It requires prompt attention. Contact your doctor and don't wait to see if it happens a second time!

Heart Dart #3: Phlebitis

Just as arteries are at risk as you age, veins, too, can become blocked, stretched, and stiff. They are thinner than your thick, muscular arteries, and instead of relying on pressure to pump the blood through your body, they depend on surrounding muscles—as well as a complicated network of one-way valves—to move the oxygen-depleted blood along.

The veins—and, in particular, these valves—can be damaged by vascular disease. In this condition, vein walls are stretched and pulled apart so that valves cannot open or close properly. Blood has a hard time moving through these damaged veins back to the heart. If the veins become blocked, this, too, can prevent proper blood flow.

When a vein becomes inflamed, the result is called phlebitis—which literally means inflammation of the veins. Phlebitis is a condition in which a blood clot, or thrombosis, blossoms at the point of inflammation. These clots can be very painful—and they can also partially or completely block the damaged vein's blood flow.

Superficial phlebitis is exactly as it sounds: at the surface. These blood clots usually occur in the legs and dissolve within days. Deep phlebitis is more dangerous; it also occurs in the legs, but much deeper. The veins affected by deep phlebitis are usually the large, important ones. Blood clots here will be bigger and pose more danger of breaking off and traveling to the lungs. Under these circumstances, the clot is termed a pulmonary embolism—which is life-threatening because it blocks off oxygen supply to the heart.

Equally dangerous in deep phlebitis is the fact that it is deadly quiet. There are relatively few symptoms, no cramping, no pain in your legs, to signal a problem.

Some of the causes of phlebitis are:

- *Varicose veins.* These bulging, bluish veins seen on the surface of your skin (most commonly in the legs), are a sign that blood is not being pumped as efficiently as it should.
- *Lengthy hospital stays.* The elderly are especially vulnerable to phlebitis if they need extended bed rest—which can affect circulation.
- *Prolonged sitting.* Long plane flights (think international) greatly increase the risk of phlebitis. Lower your risk by getting up and walk every hour and doing "pumping" exercises while seated.
- *An unhealthy lifestyle.* As with other heart conditions, obesity, sedentary habits, and cigarette smoking can all increase your risk of the blood clots that come with phlebitis.
- *Diabetes.* At first glance, it doesn't seem that diabetes, a hormonal disease that impairs the body's ability to control sugar in the blood, would have anything to do with the heart. But anything in the blood—whether it's excess sugar, plaque, or fatty deposits—can affect blood flow and circulation. (Diabetes has also been found to increase the development of atherosclerosis.)

BEWARE OF THE COLD

Cold weather is not pleasant for anyone, but for those in their senior years, it can be particularly dangerous. Not only can the ice and cold cause falls, breathing problems, and chapped, raw skin, but hypothermia as well. Any substantial drop in body temperature below the normal range of 98° can cause an irregular heartbeat and, ultimately, heart failure. What's particularly risky about hypothermia is that it is not always caused by a blast of cold air. It can result from extended illness or certain medications that inhibit your body's ability to regulate its internal temperature.

If you or someone you love is very cold, sleepy and confused, weak, shivering, or slurring speech, get out of the cold and into a hospital—immediately!

Heart Dart #4: Atrial Fibrillation

No, this is not a geographical location. Nor is it a new dance or an on-the-edge rock group. (Although it would make a great question for the newest prime time game show!)

Atrial fibrillation is actually an irregular heartbeat that can occur as you age. Your heart pumps blood through your body in a rhythmic burst of blood. Put your finger at your pulse on the inside of your wrist. Every beat you feel is a rhythmic surge of blood being pushed through your bloodstream.

Your heart is an extremely efficient machine. The burst of blood at every beat moves in a pattern. Some of your surging blood is pushed through a valve in the atrium. Other blood is pushed out the valve of a ventricle. Still other blood passes through the aorta out into your blood stream. The rhythm and the movement of the valves are crucial for a sustained, consistent push of blood throughout your body. When that rhythm gets off kilter, so will your supply of blood.

This irregular heartbeat (atrial fibrillation) is a warning that your heart, in particular, the atrium, is not pumping blood efficiently. The dangerous result: Clots can develop within the atrium of the heart—ready to travel up to the brain and cause a stroke or to an arm or leg and cause gangrene. Learn to

LUNG SLUGS

Your lungs can have their own problems—ones which have nothing to do with the heart. They can hamper your lifestyle as you age, particularly in the form of asthma.

Although children are especially susceptible to asthma, it is being discovered in many women after menopause—and the numbers are rising. Brought on by allergies—particularly animal dander and pollen, stress, or bronchitis—asthma is an inflammation of the trachea and bronchioles in the lungs which causes swelling; a person having an attack cannot breathe out. Airways become clogged with mucus and stale air gets trapped in the lungs. You begin to wheeze, trying to exhale. Eventually, the swollen airways become so narrow that no air can be passed in or out. Inhalers containing a variety of medications can be used to open up the lung's constricted airways and reduce the number of attacks. Steroids, available as both tablets and inhalers, can help prevent attacks from taking place.

take your pulse and check for an irregular heartbeat. Your doctor can confirm if your heart needs treatment.

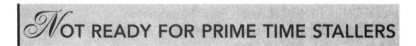

$\mathcal{N}$OT READY FOR PRIME TIME STALLERS

Now that you know all the things that can happen to your heart, the "heart darts" that can railroad a life, it's most definitely time for the good news.

And there is a great deal. Today, we know much more about the heart and how it works. We have powerful medicines and treatments to make a heart healthy again. And we also have scores of research that show exactly how a heart can remain healthy well into your golden years. We call this good news the "Heart Smarts."

Let's go over the top 10 "heart smarts" now:

Heart Smart #10: Aspirin. Yes, the ads are correct. Plain old over-the-counter aspirin is a very effective medicine for heart disease. It helps thin the blood and has been found to prevent heart attack and stroke by 25%. The recommended daily dosage varies from 325 mg (one tablet of regular-strength aspirin) to as little as 81 mg (one baby aspirin). Always check with your doctor, however, before taking aspirin. It may cause bleeding, especially in people with high blood pressure.

Pentoxifylline, one of the first "blood thinners" after aspirin, introduced in 1972, has other uses. Although not specifically used for heart conditions, it can improve blood circulation in your extremities, improving blood flow and pain from leg cramping. Its brand name is Trental®. The newest blood-thinner available today is called Pletal® and it may provide even better protection.

Heart Smart #9: Anticoagulants. Although people think this group of drugs also thins the blood, that's not quite right. Actually, anticoagulants prevent blood clots from forming in the arteries and veins. But their protection doesn't come without risk. (The common anticoagulant Coumadin®, for example, is a rat poison in higher dosages!) Anticoagulants can also cause internal bleeding (hemorrhaging).

But, under a doctor's care, anticogulants can do a tremendous amount of good. For example, one study found that Coumadin® can reduce the risk of stroke in patients over 65 with atrial fibrillation by approximately 66%. This is particularly important since atrial fibrillation increases dramatically with age; learn how to take your pulse and recognize the beats of atrial fibrillation.

Still other studies show that anticoagulants are successful in preventing second strokes in people who have had embolic strokes (in which a blood clot travels to the brain).

Other studies, however, have found that anticoagulants are less effective in preventing transient ischemic attacks (the "mini strokes" that act as warning signs. Heparin® is usually administered in a hospital, directly into a vein. When a patient leaves the hospital, she is usually given Coumadin®, which is taken orally at home.

Heart Smart #8: Vitamin E and Other Antioxidants. There's been a lot of talk in the media about antioxidants; these powerful substances are supposed to do everything from stopping the aging process to preventing cancer to keeping your skin wrinkle free. What an antioxidant actually does is to stop free radicals (toxic chemical by-products from foods and the environment) from invading our cells. Antioxidants "cling" to free radical molecules and prevent them from doing damage. Antioxidants also help keep our hearts healthy—and one of the most potent of these is vitamin E. Studies have found that taking 400 to 600 mg of vitamin E a day can help reduce atherosclerosis and reduce the risk of heart disease.

Studies have also found that taking folic acid and vitamin B6, two other powerful supplements found in every multivitamin on the market, helps decrease levels of homocysteine in the blood. An amino acid by-product, homocysteine—along with high blood pressure and cholesterol—is one of the most common culprits behind the plaque that clings to and weakens artery walls. The Physician's Health Study at Harvard found that 95% of the people in the study who had heart disease had high levels of homocysteine. Folic acid and vitamin B6 convert potentially harmful homocysteine into the benign cysteine.

Heart Smart #7: Digitalis Medications. Digitalis was the "original" natural remedy. First obtained from the flowering plant foxglove, it is now synthetically made in the laboratory where potency can be more readily supervised. Used for congestive heart failure and atrial fibrillation, digitalis helps strengthen the heart and restore correct rhythm. Side effects include nausea, headaches, fatigue, and digestive problems.

Digitalis should always be taken under the supervision of a physician because it poses several risks. It must never be stopped abruptly; it is easy to overdose on digitalis; it can also cause a reaction if taken with certain other medications, including antacids, anti-diarrheal drugs, diuretics, and certain antibiotics. Despite these risks, however, digitalis can be a real lifesaver. It's brand name is Lanoxin®.

Heart Smart #6: Nitroglycerine. This drug has been around since the late 19th century—1847 to be exact! Nitroglycerine, a vasodilator, can successfully relieve acute pain in the chest during angina episodes by making the blood vessels relax and "open" so that blood can more easily flow through your arteries. It can also work as a preventive for angina, as well as congestive heart failure and recurrent heart attack. Nitroglycerine is most commonly taken in pill form—underneath the tongue where it dissolves; it can be taken several times a day. (This is called sublingual). It is also prescribed in patch form (which research shows may not be as effective in the long-run), ointments, sprays, and long-acting pills that are swallowed.

Heart Smart #5: Antihypertensives. High blood pressure can be a thing of the past. It can be controlled to the point where it doesn't exist—as long as you lead a healthy lifestyle and keep taking your high blood pressure pills (along with the 40 million other Americans who are currently taking them). Antihypertensive medications work in several different ways: They can be a diuretic; a calcium channel blocker; an angiotensin-converting enzyme (ACE) inhibitor; or a sympathetic nerve inhibitor which blocks the brain's ability to tell the arteries to constrict. The type of medication your physician decides to give you depends on how severe your blood pressure is, as well as the other medications you might be taking, and, most importantly, which ones are effective for you. Some of the more common antihyperintensives include Vasotec®, Cardizem®, beta blockers, hydrochlorothiazide, and verapamil.

Finally, you don't need a prescription to restrict the salt in your diet—one of the most important but underutilized treatments for hypertension. Read labels. If you have high blood pressure, try to keep your salt intake around 3000 mg per day. And please note: Many of those "healthy" quick meals are loaded with salt that can make your blood pressure soar.

Heart Smart #4: Cholesterol-Reducing Drugs. Although nothing can replace the benefits of a healthy diet, low in saturated fats (a common root of high cholesterol), these fairly new drugs can reduce the amount of LDL or "bad" cholesterol in your arteries and raise the vacuum-cleaning HDL or "good" cholesterol. Some work by inhibiting production of total cholesterol; others break down and destroy deposits on arterial walls. Side effects may include dizziness, nausea, headache, stomach cramps, and muscle aches. Cholesterol-reducing drugs can also counter interact with certain medications, especially anticoagulants.

Some of the most popular cholesterol-reducing drugs are in the group called the "statins": lovastatin, pravastatin, and simvastatin. These medications are HMG-CoA reductase inhibitors, which is a technical way of saying that they alter levels of blood fat and cholesterol by blocking an enzyme in the liver that is needed for cholesterol to be produced in the first place. Less

enzyme, less cholesterol. Statins also increase the levels of HDL in the bloodstream. If your physician prescribes a statin, make sure to let her know about other medications you may be taking. Statins can interact adversely with certain antibiotics, immune-suppression medications, and niacin. Further, you should not drink grapefruit juice if you are taking any statin drugs. Grapefruit juice triggers your body to metabolize these medications too quickly and you can get a toxic reaction.

Heart Smart #3: Interventional Procedures.   When medication fails, a variety of procedures today can be extremely successful. David Letterman, for example, had quadruple bypass surgery and, one month later, was hosting his *Late Show* again.

The most common procedure today is balloon angioplasty. Technically, a nonsurgical technique, angioplasty involves placing a catheter in a blocked artery to restore blood flow; the catheter is inserted in the body either at the arm or groin, then threaded up to the blocked artery. At the tip of the catheter is a deflated balloon—which is inflated during the procedure. As it expands, the balloon pushes through and breaks up the blockage in the artery, allowing normal flow. The doctor may also insert a frame-like holding, called a *stent*, to keep the artery open long after the ballooning has done its work. Some doctors are using lasers in a "roto rooter" fashion to break up thick atherosclerotic plaque.

Bypass surgery is much more complicated and is usually done when the blocked blood vessel cannot be treated by angioplasty. With the use of a piece of vein from the leg, thigh, foot, or internal mammary artery as a new vessel, blood is actually rerouted around the blocked artery. The blocked artery is, as the surgery suggests, bypassed. Coronary bypass surgery can significantly increase both the quality and length of a person's life.

Heart Smart #2: Know the Signs.   Some symptoms of a heart attack are unmistakable: a crushing pain in the chest; a shooting pain on the left side of your body, radiating out from your shoulder and down your arm; heavy sweating; nausea; and clammy, pale skin. Other symptoms, however, are much less obvious, especially in women. These include indigestion, nausea, heart palpitations, shortness of breath, fluid retention, lightheadedness, and dizziness. Of course, none of these symptoms by themselves may be serious, but if you have any sense that you are not feeling well, get to a hospital. The worst you'll feel is embarrassed. Remember to have your blood pressure checked regularly, especially if you are at risk,

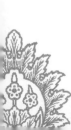

and to schedule yearly physicals. Knowledge will surely make you "heart smart."

And, finally, (drum roll, please), our number one prevention solution for heart disease.

Heart Smart #1: Maintain a Healthy Lifestyle. Most of the risk factors associated with heart disease involve habits—which you can change. A sedentary lifestyle. Obesity. Cigarette smoking. Stress. These are all factors that you can control. More than anything else, you can help prevent heart disease by living a healthy life style. This includes:

* *Eating a low-fat diet.* Saturated fats, like butter and trans fatty acids found in margarine, can contribute to cholesterol build-up.
* *Exercising regularly.* Join a gym. Take a walk. Become active in your daily life and schedule definite time for activity.
* *Practicing stress reduction.* Through meditation, yoga, or deep breathing exercises.
* *Quitting smoking.* We don't have to say any more about tobacco. You know the score.
* *Getting a good night's sleep.* You need time to rewind and for your body to replenish itself.
* *Keeping a positive outlook.* It will not only help you enjoy life more, but being positive has also been found to reduce blood pressure.

For more information about heart disease, contact:

American Heart Association
7272 Greenville Avenue
Dallas, TX 75231-4596
(214) 373-6300
(800) AHA-USA1
(214) 706-1341 (fax)
www.amhrt.org

**American Heart, Lung, and Blood Institute
   Information Center**
P. O. Box 30105
Bethesda, MD 20824-0105
(800) 575-WELL
(301) 251-1223 (fax)
E-mail: nhibiic@DGS.dgsys.com
www.gek.best.vwh.net

American Lung Association
1740 Broadway
New York, NY 10019-4374
(212) 315-8700
(212) 265-5642 (fax)
www.lungusa.org

American Dietetic Association
216 W. Jackson Boulevard, Suite 800
Chicago, IL 60606
(800) 366-1655
www.eatright.org

We've spent a great deal of time inside your "house." Let's get some fresh air—and walk out the door to the front yard, where we'll be examining skin problems next.

THE FRONT YARD: SKIN PROBLEMS

Do not be anxious about tomorrow; tomorrow will look after itself.
—Matthew 6:34

It was something Sue regretted now with all her heart, but it was too late—or so she thought. When Sue was a teenager, she liked nothing more than sitting in the sun. She spent vacations slathered in oil by the pool from early morning until late afternoon. Weekends meant blaring radios, chaise lounges, and tanning oil in the backyard.

Sue didn't swim, except to cool off. She didn't sail. She didn't read. She didn't play Frisbee. All Sue did was sit in the sun. She loved her tan; it brought out the blue in her eyes and made her hair even blonder. She'd wear white bathing suits to emphasize her golden color.

She was methodical about it: One hour on each side. She basted herself with oil as if she were a chicken.

Forty years later, she looked like a chicken. Her face was leathery and wrinkled; she had brown spots on her hands and chest. She no longer looked like a bathing beauty.

Now that Sue was in her 50s, she was very careful about the sun. She'd read the reports about skin cancer and she was scared. She slathered on sunscreen; she used Renova®, a Retin-A® product, to try to minimize her wrinkles. And she went to her dermatologist twice a year to make sure she was free of skin cancer.

Although Sue was lucky so far, she was not satisfied. The vanity of her teenage years had not gone away; it had just changed its form. Sue became obsessed with the idea of cosmetic surgery. She wanted to do something, anything, to get rid of her leathery skin.

Her doctor suggested a chemical peel, a procedure in which the damaged surface layer of skin is removed. It wasn't too expensive, but it required several visits. Sue agreed. It would be worth it if her skin looked better.

For three months, Sue went through "vanity hell." Her skin burned; she looked red and blotchy. But, once her face had healed, she noticed a softer look. Her lines were less noticeable. Her skin actually had a pink tone.

Sue was thankful that she lived in a world where so many options were available. She doesn't go near the water anymore— unless she has a hat and a wide beach umbrella. She lectures her family and friends on the perils of the sun. And she is very, very careful; she never misses her dermatologist appointments.

Sue couldn't go back in time and change years of a damaging habit, but she could do something now and in the future. And that, along with her cheeks, is looking rosy indeed.

When we think of aging and the skin, we tend to feel superficial, that it's all a matter of vanity. But, in reality, skin is more than, well, skin deep. Feeling good about our appearances helps us feel good about our circumstances. It gives us confidence and helps reduce our stress—which ultimately helps keep our minds and bodies healthy and sound.

In addition to being the "façade" we show the world, skin is an important organ. It acts like a shield, a barrier, from the world at large; it protects us.

But sometimes skin breaks down. It gets tired, blotchy, saggy. You may have a cancerous mole. (Skin cancer is one of the most common cancers today.) *But skin cancer can be totally eradicated if caught early enough.*

That fact alone would give skin its own "room" in your "house." But skin is an outer organ. And because it is so important to our health and our psyche, it gets the whole front yard. Let's go outside and get "under your skin."

SKIN ALIVE

The skin, or cutis, is the "fence" that keeps external infections, temperatures, and stimulation at bay. It protects our muscles, bones, blood vessels, nerves, and organs. It's quite a job! It makes sense that skin, although it looks as if it's just one tough piece, is really a complicated combination of three distinct, "skin deep" layers that, together, are called (for all you trivia buffs or quiz show contestant hopefuls) the integumentary system.

Skin Deep #1: Epidermis

This is the skin we show the world and, although we may buff it, clean it, and enhance it, this outer layer is really a layer of dead cells called *squamous*.

These cells don't start out dead. At the point where the epidermis meets the second layer, the dermis, there is a "rug" of basal cells. These plump cells are a lifeline to the bloodstream. But, unlike the soft pile rugs on your floors, this layer of basal cells is rigid. As more cells are produced, the older basal cells are pushed off the "rug." Without their lifeline, they die and become squamous cells. As more and more new cells are produced on the basal "rug," more and more squamous cells are pushed up and out. Eventually, they flake off. In fact, we lose approximately 500 million squamous cells a day—and 500 million new basal cells are produced to take their place. As we shower and dress, scratch an itch and rub on lotion, our skin is literally alive with this flaking off activity.

The dead squamous cells are flat, flaky, and fibrous from a hard material called keratin. Despite their hard, dead composition, these squamous cells form a layer of skin that can stretch and pull as you gain or lose weight, and as you move about. As you age, this stretchy layer of skin loses some its firmness. It doesn't bounce back as easily. The keratin also builds up, creating tough, hard skin, especially on your feet and around your nails.

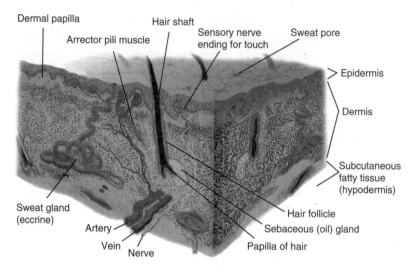

Dermal papilla

Hair shaft

Arrector pili muscle

Sensory nerve
ending for touch

Sweat pore

Epidermis

Dermis

Subcutaneous
fatty tissue
(hypodermis)

Sweat gland
(eccrine)

Artery

Vein

Nerve

Hair follicle

Sebaceous (oil) gland

Papilla of hair

Figure 15–1   Drawing of the integumentary system layers

Skin Deep #2: Dermis

Directly below the "rug" of basal cells is the layer of skin called the *dermis*. This is the "heart center" of skin, where:

- Nerve receptors register such sensations as "hot," "cold," and "tingly"
- Sweat glands, crucial for regulating body temperature, make their home
- Hair follicles begin
- Embedded nerve receptors called pacinian corpuscles reside—where they send word of deep pressure (as in a massage) to the brain

Collagen and elastin, the fibrous connective tissues that keep skin supple, are also produced in the dermis.

Skin Deep #3: Subcutaneous layer

Here's the bane of every dieter's existence, the layer of insulation that further protects the organs below the skin. The primary insulation used? Adipose tissue, or, as we hate to call it, fat.

$\mathscr{S}$KINNY DEEP

Because skin is "out there," it is the part of our body that shows aging in a most literal sense. We can keep our hearts strong with exercise, our gastrointestinal tracts smooth with a healthy diet, our brains sharp with mental stimulation. But skin? When it sags, the world can't help but see it, warts and all.

Here are some of the ways aging landscapes our "front yard" skin—and why:

Skinful Truth #1: Gravity

The fact is that gravity eventually pulls everything down—and that includes your skin. A woman in her 20s, for example, will be in proportion; she will have pretty much the same size forehead, nose, cheeks, and chin. But, as she enters middle age, gravity begins to do its work on earlobes, chins, necks, and noses. The lower half of the face is particular vulnerable to the effects of gravity—which is why face-lifts are so popular.

Short of becoming an astronaut, there's not much you can do to prevent gravity's pull. But exercise and maintaining a consistent weight help keep your skin toned and firm.

Skinful Truth #2: Sun exposure

You know the pitfalls of this one. In fact, in today's health-conscious world, tans are out. Pale skin and self-bronzers are in. But unless you spent your entire life living under a hat and slathered in sunscreen, your skin will show some effects of decades of sun.

When the radiation from the sun's rays hits your skin, it enters the nucleus, or center, of your skin cells, damaging the cells so much over time that they can no longer produce the skin's "fountain of youth"—fibrous collagen and elastin. These fibers keep your skin supple, glowing, and wrinkle-free. Over time, as your skin produces less and less of these fibers, wrinkles crop up. Skin becomes leathery. And damage to the nuclei of the cells can become so severe that the cells become cancerous.

THE KILLER BOOTH

John Wilkes Booth, the man who assassinated President Lincoln, wasn't the only "killer." Tanning *booths* can also be dangerous. They utilize UVA rays which may increase the risk of the skin cancer called melanoma by increasing the number of melanocytes in your body. Proceed with caution! Tanning beds are no safer than the sun and can be extremely dangerous.

There are two types of ultraviolet radiation from the rays of the sun that cause problems. UVB rays are the most aggressive; they cause burning and subsequent damage. UVA rays are shorter; they don't burn skin so protection from them is not always included in a sunscreen product. But UVA rays can also cause skin damage, including cancer and precancerous growths called keratoses. Always look for a product that contains both UVA/UVB protection. Dermatologists recommend sunscreens with a minimum sun protection factor (SPF) of 15.

At the very least, early sun damage will show up in later years as brown spots. They are often called "liver spots" as well because of their brown-gray color—not because there is any connection to the liver! These spots are found typically on the back of your hands, face, and chest. They are a result of excess melatonin, a pigment in the skin that makes you tan when you are exposed to the sun. Products containing hydroquinone can help them fade if the spot is near the surface of the epidermis. Photofacials®, utilizing high-energy light, are expensive but highly effective in erasing these brown spots.

Too much sun will also cause wrinkles and leathery skin in later life. This is the "photoaging" that anti-wrinkle products, such as Retin-A®, help reduce.

At its worst, sun damage can cause skin cancer in later life. Twenty years ago, only 1 in 1000 seniors got melanoma, the most severe type of skin cancer. Today that percentage has risen to 1 in 100. Obviously, people who live in warmer climates are more at risk and need to wear sunscreen at all times. Reapply thoroughly before you go out and reapply often during the day to replace the protection lost from sweating and swimming. And don't forget your sons and daughters! Start teaching them to use sunscreen early on. Much of the skin damage occurs before the age of 21.

Women are more likely to develop skin cancer than men because they tend to sit in the sun more. Fortunately, they are also more likely to notice a mole on the skin that has changed shape—a cancer warning sign.

And while we are on the subject, here' some information on the three different types of skin cancers and their warning signs. Read it. Check your skin routinely. And see your doctor if any of the signs sound familiar. Skin cancer is the most curable of all cancers—if it is caught early enough.

Basal cell carcinoma.   This is the most common type of skin cancer; it affects 1 in 6 aging baby boomers; people over 40 with fair skin are most at risk. It rarely spreads to other organs, and it is the easiest to remove. If left unattended, however, it can spread locally, causing significant disfigurement and damage. It starts as a small red bump in places where you have been exposed to the sun. Eventually, its center crusts and bleeds.

Squamous cell carcinoma.   One in 50 people develop this type of skin cancer; it is most prevalent in fair-skinned people over 60; aging baby boomers who have spent their lives in the sun are most at risk. It is more dangerous than basal cell cancer because it can spread quickly to other organs. These tumors look like small hard moles with a scaly, crusty texture. You'll find them more often on necks, hands, arms, ears, and lips.

Melanoma.   This skin cancer is the most dangerous of all because it not only moves quickly and lethally to other organs, but it is frequently fatal if not caught early enough. This tumor might start out as a mole that crops up where none existed or as a familiar mole that has become irregular in shape. It can grow wider, redden, bleed, and change shape, color, and depth. Although a melanoma is usually dark in color, it can, at times, lack its characteristic darker pigment. The best way to tell? See your physician for annual "body checks." And don't forget what you can do at home. Check your own body in the same way you examine your breasts on a monthly basis. And ask someone to check the places you can't see for potentially dangerous skin lesions.

THE PINK THAT ISN'T ROSY

Another skin condition that affects aging baby boomers is an adult acne called rosacea, which shows up on your face in tiny broken blood vessels that make your complexion ruddy and blotchy. Rosacea can also create tiny pimples, especially on your cheeks and nose. Although the condition can have genetic roots, it is more likely a result of bacteria and hormonal shifts. Alcohol, caffeine, and spicy food have also been linked to rosacea. The good news is that rosacea can be treated with antibiotics such as tetracycline, antibiotic ointments such as Metrogel® and Photofacial® reduce the redness by 60–70% in most cases. Catch it early and the results are even that much better!

Remember, skin cancer does not have to be fatal. Wearing sunscreen and going for regular check-ups can prevent skin cancer from growing. It can be removed and never come back!

Skinful Truth #3: Smoking

Just in case you needed another reason to quit smoking: It causes wrinkles. In fact, studies have found that people with the same life experiences, including age, complexion, and exposure to the sun, had more wrinkles if they smoked. In other words, if you smoke and sit in the sun, you'll end up looking older than you are. Why? Possibly because smoking hinders circulation so the flow of blood to your skin is hampered. If you combine smoking with sun over-exposure, your skin doesn't stand a chance!

Skinful Truth #4: Overheated Air

In case you haven't noticed, the older you get, the dryer your skin becomes. If you find yourself hitting the hand lotion bottle more frequently now, you're not alone. Not only do sweat and oil gland production diminish as you age, but years of using soap, bathing and showering, and applying antiperspirants and perfumes also help dry out the skin.

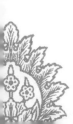

BEAUTIFUL SKIN AROUND THE WORLD AND THROUGH HISTORY

Ancient Romans knew that the sun was bad for you. Pale skin was highly prized, and women achieved the "marble statue look" with white lead and chalk.

Elizabethans in Renaissance England liked their skin glowing and pink. Women got their blushing rose by washing their face with wine.

Even today the Far East does things a little differently than us. In China, pulverized pearls are used to keep skin smooth. In Malaysia, women make homemade facials from fermented rice and water.

And what about us? Contemporary American women use everything from maple syrup, red wine grapes, Vitamin C, seaweed, and sea salt to get younger-looking skin. Indeed, cosmetic departments have practically taken over the first floor of many department stores and they even have their own stores: Sephora is a department store exclusively devoted to cosmetics.

But the biggest culprit of dry, itchy skin is overheated air. If people in sunny climes are more susceptible to sun damage, people in the north are more likely to suffer from dry, dehydrated skin. Heaters, radiators, and indoor heating units all tend to suck moisture from the air; heated air itself is very dry. If you find you put the heat up several notches in the winter, make sure you also use a humidifier to replace the moisture in the air.

RAGING AGING: THE QUEST TO MAKE SKIN BEAUTIFUL

Anti-aging creams and lotions have always had huge success in the marketplace, but their popularity has never been what it is today, as millions of aging baby boomers try to turn back the clock, remove the wrinkles and photoaging from too much sun, and make their faces glowing, soft, and supple once again.

Here are some of the "miracles" on the market today. Some of them do work amazingly well. Some are quite expensive. Others show only slight improvements on the skin—but help make you feel better about yourself. Others are a waste of money. Become an informed shopper for "what price vanity."

Miracle Potion #1: A Fruit by Any Other Name— Alpha-Hydroxy Acid (AHA) Lotions and Fruit-Enzyme Creams

These creams are the least expensive and most accessible way to go. They contain acids from fruit such as strawberry and pineapple, as well as a small percentage of an AHA acid such as Retin-A®, which, together, gently exfoliate the toughened, leathery first layer of skin. The result is smoother, more glowing skin. Because these products are sold over the counter and in cosmetic departments, the active ingredients make up only a small percentage of the total cream or lotion. They work, but they are gentle enough for anyone's skin. You'll see some slight improvement, but no "miracle."

Renova®, a form of Retin-A®—both of which contain the peeling chemical tretinoin—has been found to work better than mild, over-the-counter products. You need to get a doctor's prescription for Renova® and it costs about $60.00. A word of caution: these products can make you more sensitive to the sun. It is mandatory that you apply these products only at night and use sunscreen during the day.

A newer product, called Kinerase®, contains N6-furfuryladenine which, unlike its Renova® cousins, does not make you more sensitive to the sun. Almay® makes a line of inexpensive products containing it called Kinetin®.

Antioxidants are also making age-reducing headlines. Vitamin E, an ingredient in many alpha-hydroxy creams, helps promote skin healing and decrease scarring. Vitamin C too is being touted in many anti-aging creams. But because it can lose its potency quickly when exposed to air, make sure you are getting a product in a light-resistant, air-tight container.

Miracle Potion #2: Chemical Peels—Like Peeling a Grape

Chemical peels, done in a dermatologist's office or licensed salon, go deeper than that first, outer layer of skin. The deeper they go, the greater the improvement. Chemical peels primarily use a high percentage of glycolic acid or stronger percentage of AHA. Chemical peels done in a salon typically have an acid percentage of 30%. Stronger peels—as high as 70%—must be done by a dermatologist or cosmetic surgeon; you'll need about 6 to 10 treatments to see results. (One-time-only treatments can leave your skin red, inflamed, and painful; it is best to do the peeling gradually.)

Microdermabrasion is a powerful mechanical peel that pushes fine sand against the face under very high pressure, then immediately vacuums it back up—leaving behind smoother skin. It may work best when combined with Photofacial® or another technique that brings the pigment and damaged skin to the surface.

Miracle #3: Beam Me Young—Laser Surgery

Laser peels and surgery have an added bonus that you won't find with ordinary peels: They have been found to stimulate the skin's production of collagen—which translates into firmer, tighter, softer skin.

Laser resurfacing uses a pulsing carbon-dioxide laser on your wrinkles. It literally vaporizes several outer layers of skin, revealing the smoother, tighter, more flattened skin below. Used around the mouth, the laser is pinpointed in the areas between your wrinkles—which pulls them taut and reduces their appearance. The main side-effect? Possible dark blotches and scarring.

Photofacials® is a new non-invasive procedure. As we've mentioned earlier, it is a type of laser that uses an intense, pulsating light to tighten collagen in the skin as well as remove

I AM MAN, HEAR ME ROAR

If you think only women are interested in cosmetic surgery, think again. Men are opting for facelifts, laser surgery, peels, and lotions to the tune of $10 billion every year! Cosmetic grooming aids such as lotions, bronzers, and moisturizers for men are growing at a rate of 10% every year.

Most men don't want to take the weeks off that healing from facelifts entail. Instead, they opt for milder forms of dermabrasion and use laser procedures as their fountain of youth of choice.

excessive brown pigment and redness. The procedure takes 30 minutes, and there is no "down time." You can return to work immediately. It is expensive and requires 5 to 6 treatments, but the results have been impressive.

Whatever procedure you choose, use an experienced surgeon with excellent references to get the beautiful skin you want.

Miracle Potion #4: Facelifts—Waiting for a Lift

The ultimate miracle cure for aging, of course, is the facelift. When performed by the right hands, it can sweep away the years from your neck, chin, eyes, and cheeks. And it's no longer the province of the rich: More than 1 million people have already gone under the knife for the sake of vanity.

New procedures are less invasive than those of years past, when movie stars and other celebrities had to "hide" for months. Tiny incisions, like keyholes, are made on droopy eyelids and brows, fleshy jowls, and neck wattles through which the skin is literally lifted and tightly pulled back. There is less chance of scarring and the telltale marks at the earlobe or chin that spell facelift are non-existent. But there is still risk involved: facial nerve injury, asymmetric eyebrows, cheeks, and foreheads—not to mention infection and the risks involved in general anesthesia. It is vitally important that you use a specialist who has had much experience and many glowing recommendations—even if you have to wait for an appointment. Facelifts can cost anywhere from approximately $6,000 to over $12,000. And don't get greedy and go for too much of a good thing. Remember the women you've seen whose skin looked pulled too tight and artificial. Communicate your feelings to your surgeon.

Miracle Potion #5: Liposuction

We all know what it is—and, lately, the press on it has not been very good. The fact is that liposuction is a very basic procedure: excess body fat is "sucked out" from the body via small incisions; suction tubes are inserted into the incisions and, by moving around inside fat pockets, the fat itself is dissolved and removed. Liposuction can remove fairly large pockets of fat and give your hips and thighs a more contoured appearance. Although liposuction won't remove cellulite and it won't flatten your stomach

HAIR LOSS IS A PROBLEM FOR WOMEN, TOO

It's normal to lose up to 400 strands of hair every day, but if you notice more than your share of strands in the bathtub drain, it's possible that you have a condition called alopecia. Twenty million American women suffer from alopecia, but it can go away all by itself. Stress is one of the leading factors of hair loss; chronic anxiety can actually cause up to 30% of a woman's hair to grow prematurely from the growth stage (called anagen) to the resting stage (called telogen) when hair is shed. Once your stress is relieved, the hair will usually grow back. Hormones are also a big trigger: the loss of estrogen during menopause can cause your hair to shed. But HRT or low-dosage birth control pills can usually reverse the problem.

Rogaine® is still the only nonprescription medication that has been proven to slowly regrow hair.

(you'll need a tummy tuck or abdominoplasty for that), it can take as much as ten pounds off your bottom half. It is even done on the neck and jowls.

So why the bad press? You also lose a lot of fluid along with the fat. And, because it is often done in a doctor's office or an outpatient facility, emergency situations (such as fat emboli–clots–to the brain), may arise that need a hospital environment and can have serious consequences. Further, liposuction must be done by an experienced physician; it's crucial that you check out references and credentials before deciding to have it.

Convalescence takes several weeks, during which time you must wear a special girdle or tight stocking; this keeps swelling down, prevents bleeding, and helps shrink your skin to fit its new contours. You can expect bruising, pain, and numbness in the first few weeks. If you do not religiously exercise afterwards, all the pain, time, and money will be wasted!

A newer form of liposuction has been found to be much safer. Tumescent liposuction uses a solution of salt water, lidocaine (a local anesthetic), and blood-vessel shrinking adrenaline that is injected into the fat before the suction begins. This helps reduce pain, swelling, and bruising later on.

Lipoplasty uses ultrasonic energy to get out the fat. A sound wave probe attacks only the fat cells, breaking them up without harming any other nearby cells. The dissolved fat is then removed by suction. This process, too, helps minimize any aftereffects.

Magic Potion #6: Botox® and Other Line-Smoothing Injections

Yes, it's true. Botox® is the same ingredient found in botulism toxin. But, in the minute dosages that are used to smooth wrinkles on your forehead, around your lips, and near your eyes, it can be perfectly safe. Botox® actually weakens the muscles where it is injected, creating a smooth appearance. The treatment lasts for several months—after which time you'll need to go back for another injection. To help avoid the possibility of bruising, try to avoid using bruise-friendly aspirin, vitamin E, or alcohol a week before your treatment. Avoid rubbing the spot right after an injection; this will ensure that the Botox® doesn't spread to surrounding muscles.

Botox® is becoming very mainstream and very safe—but it should still be only administered in a physician's office and by a physician. But make sure you've checked out the physician who will be performing the procedure. This is your body after all! Botox® can cost anywhere from $325 to over $500 for each treatment.

Collagen works by "plumping up." When injected into a wrinkle, collagen "plumps" up the skin and lips so that the wrinkle virtually disappears. However, the effects of collagen only last for a few months—and people can have an allergic reaction to it. Most collagen comes from cows or human cadavers; to avoid any thought of mad cow disease or infection, scientists have developed bioengineered human collagen.

The safest "plumper upper" is your own fat. Taken from the buttocks, this fat is used as implants to shape cheekbones or, when injected, as a wrinkle filler. Since it is your own fat that's being used, there's no chance of an allergic reaction.

Look for new "fillers" on the market; there's one introduced in this country every six to eight months. Artecoll® combines bovine collagen with polmethylmethacrylate, a chemical that stimulates collagen growth in your body. Fillers containing hyaluronic acid form a nice, plump "soup" for skin cells; hyaluronic acid is found in all mammals.

For more information about your skin and anti-aging procedures, contact:

National Institute of Arthritis and Musculoskeletal and Skin Diseases (NIAMS) Clearinghouse
1 AMS Circle
Bethesda, MD 20892-3675
(301) 495-4484
www.hiams.nih.gov/hi/

National Cancer Institute (NCI)
9000 Rockville Pike
Building 31, Room 10A24
Bethesda, MD 20892
(800) 4-CANCER
www.nci.nih.gov

The Skin Cancer Foundation
245 Fifth Avenue, Suite 2402
New York, NY 10016
(800) SKIN-490
(212) 725-5176
(212) 725-5751 (fax)
www.skincancer.org

American Board of Medical Specialities
1007 Church Street, Suite 404
Evanston, IL 60201
(800) 776-CERT
(Provides information on board certified cosmetic surgeons and dermatologists)
www.abms.org

American Academy of Dermatology
P.O. Box 4014
Schaumburg, IL 60168-4014
(847) 330-0230
(847) 330-0050 (fax)
www.aad.org

This ends our break outside. It's time to stop tending our front yard and visit the last, and one of the most popular, rooms in your "house": the kitchen—where you'll discover your body's gastrointestinal tract and the problems that can arise—and be treated—as you age.

CHAPTER

16

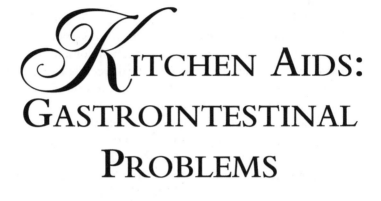

KITCHEN AIDS: GASTROINTESTINAL PROBLEMS

If you can't make it better, you can laugh at it.
—Erma Bombeck

Caroline woke up with a start. She doubled over in pain. Sure that she was having a heart attack, she woke her husband. But before he could even call an ambulance, the pain was gone. Caroline felt a little nauseous and weak, but other than that, she felt fine.

She decided instead to call her doctor the next day. But in the morning, Caroline felt wonderful. There were no aftereffects from her awful night. Besides, she had a big presentation at work that afternoon. And she and her husband were going to see their teenage daughter in her high school play that evening.

In short, Caroline forgot all about her attack. Although her husband suggested she call the doctor, Caroline seemed fine. He stopped reminding her; he didn't want to be a nag.

Several weeks later, the same thing happened again—this time at a Thanksgiving dinner at her in-law's house. Caroline had just had a huge meal—turkey, gravy, and all the fixings. She had piled on the pie and ice cream, and she had had to unbutton her skirt.

She was sitting in the living room, watching the game with her family, when the pain struck. It was a sharp, sudden stab in her upper torso. Caroline felt nauseous; she started to shiver; she needed to throw up.

Then, as suddenly as it had started, the pain subsided. This time, however, her husband wasn't going to let the incident slide. Together, they left the party and went to the emergency room.

After the doctor probed Caroline's abdomen and asked her questions about her diet and what she'd recently eaten, he gave his diagnosis: gallstones. He ordered an ultrasound of Caroline's abdomen and gallbladder to remove any doubt.

Gallstones? That only happened to old people, Caroline insisted. And she was only 51. That wasn't old! Gallstones were the province of her mother; she had had gallstones. She remembered going over to her mother's house to take her out to dinner, only to find her in the bathroom feeling sick with cramps and nausea.

But Caroline couldn't deny the evidence. She ate a lot of fat—and very little roughage. The doctor believed her gallstones had been floating around in her gallbladder for 20 years, growing with every high-fat meal she ate. The reason for the sudden symptoms was that a stone had moved from her gallbladder into the narrow bile duct leading to her intestine.

The stone eventually —and painfully—"passed" on its own so Caroline didn't require surgery. But she did have to change her ways. She had to eat a healthier diet; she didn't have to eliminate fat completely, but she had to eat fewer of those desserts and fried foods. She also needed to eat more fiber: fruit and vegetables as well as bran cereals.

Caroline had to learn a hard truth: Years of bad habits eventually creep up on you. Many of the physical problems aging baby boomers face are a result of an unhealthy lifestyle—problems which cannot only be prevented in youth, but in the "golden years" as well. Today, three months after her last attack, Caroline feels better than ever. She has more energy, more sparkle in her eyes, and she appreciates the foods she eats much more. She sleeps like a baby at night.

Gastrointestinal problems are extremely common, especially in seniors. Hormonal changes, medication side effects, years of poor eating habits and stress—all these can take their toll.

But before you can find ways to improve your "kitchen," you have to know where everything is.

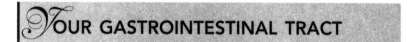 YOUR GASTROINTESTINAL TRACT

Take an apple from the fridge. Bite into it. As soon as the apple hits your mouth, your teeth chew it into tiny pieces. These pieces are further liquefied by the saliva in your mouth. The carbohydrates in the apple begin to be broken down. The process of digestion has begun.

Your tongue gets into the act, pushing the pieces of liquidy apple down past your pharynx. To prevent food from going up your nose, the soft palate at the back of your pharynx closes up your nasal cavities. A small flap called the epiglottis closes off your trachea to ensure that the apple won't go into your lungs.

The apple has only one place to go: your esophagus. This long tube is what connects your mouth to your stomach. A valve called the lower esophageal, located right above your stomach, opens and closes to allow food through.

Once this apple piece, still being broken down by enzymes and digestive juices, passes through the "guardian" sphincter, it is allowed to move down into the stomach. Here, stomach acids and enzymes such as pepsin, further break it down; at this point, it's unrecognizable. In fact, it has another name: chyme, or semi-digested food.

From the stomach, the apple-chyme goes into the upper portion of the small intestine, or the duodenum. Here, it really gets a hit from the digestive process. Fat-dissolving bile from the gallbladder and the liver pour onto the apple-chyme, and digestive enzymes from the pancreas break it down into its simplest form of nutrients—proteins into amino acids, carbohydrates into glucose, the simple sugar which is the food your body cells eat.

The broken-down apple-nutrients continue down the small intestine, into its two farthest regions: the jejunum and the ileum. By the time the original bite of apple reaches the ileum, tiny

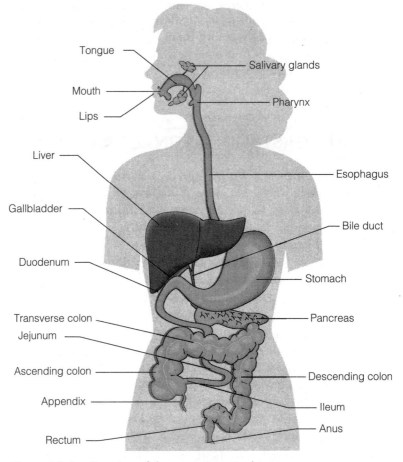

Figure 16–1 Drawing of the gastrointestinal tract

blood vessels have taken all the nutrients to the cells of your body, and only waste is left behind. This waste travels to the large intestine, where the colon, or large intestine, continues breaking it down to get any vitamins the small intestine might have missed. The water in the once-upon-a-time apple also passes through the colon walls into the bloodstream. The remaining waste, now semisolid, travels to the rectum where it is stored. Eventually, it is eliminated out the anus as feces.

Simple, orderly, and functional—until something goes awry. Years of eating—of digesting food and eliminating waste—can take its toll on our gastrointestinal tract. Here are some of the culprits, or "gut ruts," behind your cramps, gas, and discomfort:

Gut Rut #1: Blame it on the Drugs

No, this is not a part of a "Just Say No" campaign (although you should!). This gastrointestinal tract "gut wrencher" is all about the medications you take, especially as you age. Americans spend twice as much money on medications between the ages of 55 and 64 as they do in their 40s—and this amount of medicine has to have an effect on the linings of your gastrointestinal tract. High blood pressure medicine, for example, can cause constipation. So, too, can anti-anxiety drugs.

Then there are the medicines you take for gastrointestinal upsets—which can have their own set of side effects. Antacids, for example, reduce the potency of antibiotics such as tetracycline, certain heart medications such as digoxin, and iron pills prescribed for anemia. Antacids also increase the potency of tranquilizers.

The best solution? Speak to your doctor and let her know exactly what you are taking and why. She will help you establish the right dosages and make sure the medications are working with—not against—each other.

Gut Rut #2: Mucous is not just for Noses

As it does for every other organ in your body, mucous helps lubricate your gastrointestinal tract, helping food have a "smooth move" through your entire gut. But, as you age, blood flow to the gastrointestinal tract isn't as efficient as it once was. This reduction in arterial blood can create problems within the mucous linings of your gut. If your intestines become irritated, you may experience cramps, irregularity, acidity, gas, and diarrhea.

Although you can't change your age, you can change the health of your gastrointestinal tract—by eating a healthy diet, one that's high in fiber and low in fat.

Gut Rut #3: That Hormone Thing

The hormonal changes that occur as you age can also affect your gut. The cells lining the stomach and intestinal walls can erode. Some cells—in particular, gastric and small and large intestine cells—will begin to proliferate as your hormone levels change. This fast, new cell proliferation is the culprit behind the pain of gastritis; it affects the connective tissue in the gut, or the protective lining of the intestinal walls.

In short, your cells change as your hormones do. Add a poor diet, and the gut will become very susceptible to such diseases as diverticulitis, an inflammation of small pouches in the walls of the small intestine.

Gut Rut #4: A Bacteria Named Helicobacter Pylori

The bacteria Helicobacter pylori is present in the digestive tracts of many people with no ill affect. But in combination with inefficient mucus production and cell degeneration, the bacteria can blossom, crowding out stomach acids—and leaving you with a stomach ulcer. People used to think that ulcers were the product of stress and a "workaholic" lifestyle. Now we know better. If you experience pain after you've eaten, see your doctor. A regimen of antibiotics will destroy the *H. pylori* problem—and your ulcer pain.

Gut Rut #5: Enzyme Action—Lactase and Lactose

A full head of hair is not the only thing you'll lose as you age. The enzyme called lactase is another; it breaks down the lactose found in milk and dairy products. Lactose—essentially the sugar found in milk—is necessary for babies, but not for adults. It can gradually disappear as you age, causing a condition called lactose intolerance. The result is gas, acidity, and cramps after you eat or drink a dairy product.

Using lactose-free products can circumvent this condition. An over-the-counter medication designed for this problem, Lactaid®, can also help ease your discomfort.

Gut Rut #6: Jack Sprat Could Eat No Fat

Sure, you've heard this one before, but it's important enough to say again: an unhealthy diet will play havoc on your gut. Too much fat, from saturated fats, red meat, cheese, butter, and fried foods, puts your gastrointestinal tract on overload. It just can't break down the fat as efficiently as it should—especially as you age, when your tract is not operating at 100% capacity to begin with!

The result can be, as with Caroline earlier in this chapter, painful gallstones—which are nothing more than deposits of fat and cholesterol. Too much fat can also settle into pockets in the intestinal walls; if they get infected or inflamed, you can develop diverticulitis. Other conditions, too, are related to too much fat—and too little fiber: irritable bowel syndrome, gas, and constipation.

The best treatment is a simple one: go easy on the fat and pile on the fiber when you eat.

Gut Rut #7: Emotional Agenda

There's a whole group of nerves surrounding your gastrointestinal tract; they even have their own name: the enteric nervous system. You might not have heard of them, but, believe it or not, there are as many nerves here as there are in your spinal cord! When you get nervous, anxious, or upset, your brain shoots the emotions down to the enteric nerves where they are translated into queasiness and nausea—the old "butterflies in the stomach" syndrome you feel before a meeting, meeting a new beau, or going out on the stage. Stress on the enteric nervous system can also affect the rate at which food moves down your gut—resulting in diarrhea or constipation.

Reducing stress works on your gut as well as your psyche. Meditation, a leisurely walk, a warm bath, exercise—these can all help reduce emotional distress, and stomach pain.

$\mathscr{S}$TOMACH PAIN BY ANY OTHER NAME

Now that you know some of the "gut ruts" behind your growing discomfort, you can better identify the conditions they can cause. Here are the most common gastrointestinal ailments that affect aging Baby Boomers—and what you can do about them:

Don't Gotta Get a GERD

No, this is not the famous stuffed toy. GERD stands for Gastro Esophageal Reflux Disorder and, although not life-threatening, it can affect your quality of life.

Basically, GERD is heartburn, the acidic feeling you can have after eating a rich meal or when you eat on the run, on the go, and on a stressful fast track. The muscles that push the food down and keep it down in the stomach become lax as you age; acid reflux occurs when the stomach acids that flow during digestion seep back up into the esophagus and irritate its lining. Medications such as Tums® can help ease the pain, but antacids can affect other medications you are taking. There are newer over-the-counter medications out on the market now such as Pepcid® and Zantac®, but sometimes it takes a prescription medication, such as Prilosec®, Prevacid®, or Protonix®, to do the job. Ask your doctor about what's best for you.

That (Very) Irritable Bowel Syndrome (IBS)

IBS is exactly as it sounds: an irritable bowel, a condition that will make you bloated and give you painful cramps, constipation, and diarrhea, usually after you've eaten. Either you need to run to a bathroom or you just can't seem to go for the days, weeks, or months while the episode lasts, you feel as if you have no control over your gastrointestinal tract.

If this sounds familiar, you are not alone. Forty percent of all visits to gastroenterologists—doctors who specialize in the gastrointestinal (GI) tract—are because of IBS. It is the most common of all GI disorders.

Food is pushed through the intestines via peristalsis, contractions that occur in a methodical and orderly fashion. In periods of stress, however, or if your diet is high in fat, peristalsis can become irregular. This creates IBS.

The usual treatment for IBS is medication in combination with changes of diet and lifestyle. Some of the treatments your doctor may recommend:

- Staying away from fatty, greasy foods.
- Taking a bulk-forming fiber product containing psyllium.
- Taking the prescription drug loperamide to slow peristalsis.
- Taking either dicyclomine, atropine, or belladonna to ease cramps.
- Making time for stress-reducing strategies such as yoga.
- Starting a walking regimen or any other aerobic exercise. ·
- Making sure you are not lactose intolerant.
- Getting a medical exam and blood test to rule out "bile salt" diarrhea.

Those Galling Gallstones

Like Caroline at the beginning of this chapter, if you experience a sudden stab of pain a few hours after you've eaten a rich meal, it's possible that you have gallstones.

These tiny little "evil" crystal-like deposits are born in the gallbladder, the pear-shaped organ that stores bile. As the food you eat is digested, your gallbladder releases bile. This liquid, made in the liver from cholesterol and acids, travels down the cystic duct to the common bile duct where it joins forces with pancreatic juices to digest food in the small intestine.

Most of the time, the bile in the gallbladder stays liquid. In this form it moves easily from gallbladder "storage" through the cystic and common bile ducts to the small intestines without a hitch. But if you eat a lot of foods that are high in fat, the ratio of cholesterol in the bile becomes unbalanced. When the concentration becomes too heavy for the acids to dissolve, the cholesterol crystallizes into stones.

You can have several gallstones floating around in your gallbladder—and never know it. That sudden stab of pain won't occur unless the stone floats out of the roomy gallbladder and gets lodged in the narrow cystic duct.

Gallstones often pass by themselves and if the symptoms disappear, you won't have to do anything more than change your

MODERATION IN ALL THINGS

That's what the ancient Greeks said, and, in many ways, they have been proven right through the centuries ever since. Take fat, for example. Too much fat can create gallstones. But too little fat can also do the job. If you don't eat enough fat, the bile stored in the gallbladder just sits there and does nothing. The result? Lots of time for the cholesterol in the bile to build up and crystallize.

The best solution is to eat a daily diet that contains 30% fat—not too little and certainly not too much.

diet (to make sure you don't get them back!) But, if you have several episodes, your doctor may prescribe bile salt tablets to dissolve the stones, or use high-frequency sound waves to break them into fragments.

If neither of these treatments works, your doctor may insert a catheter containing a stone-dissolving drug into your abdomen. The medication will usually dissolve the stones within a few hours.

If all else fails, the gallbladder can be removed surgically. Today, that no longer means a long, difficult recuperation. Thanks to a procedure called a laparoscopic cholecystectomy, a very thin instrument is inserted and used to remove the gallbladder. With no large incision to heal, the result is a hospital stay of no more than two or three days, and considerably less pain than more traditional gallbladder operations.

Classical Gas

Belching might have been the funniest thing alive when you were 10, but as a middle-aged adult, it's no laughing matter—especially because, as an aging baby boomer, you'll be belching a lot more than your kids.

Although a burp can be the result of gallstones, stomach acid, or intestinal distress, it's usually caused by gas. The air that you swallow along with your food—usually about one-third of an ounce—usually passes out of the digestive tract without you ever noticing a thing. Gas (from that swallowed air) is, in fact, quite normal. Most people belch or flatulate at least ten times a day.

As you get older, however, your body is less efficient in passing gas. More and more air stays in the stomach or the esophagus—and it comes back up as a belch. Gas can also be caused by nervousness, too much soda, and too much gum chewing.

Another reason for gas: Eating beans and other gas-producing foods such as high-fiber vegetables and grains. Beans are not easily digested; a lot of bacterial action is needed to dissolve and metabolize them. All this work creates a by-product: gas.

The best treatments for gas are:

- Easing slowly into a high-fiber diet to get your body used to the extra digestive work.
- Seeing your doctor to make sure your gas is not a symptom of some other condition such as gallstones, lactose intolerance, or hiatal hernia.

AN OUNCE OF PREVENTION

Occult, or unseen bleeding, is the number-one symptom of colon cancer. It can be detected during a routine office visit as well as from the take-home hemoccult test. This is a card with room for three samples of stool; the laboratory will be able to determine if they contain any "invisible" blood.

If you are over 50, it is wise to do the take-home test, and have either a sigmoidoscopy or colonoscopy performed as well. Both tests involve inserting an endoscope (a tube with a light at its end) into the rectum and the large intestines. The endoscope helps the doctor see whether you have any polyps, or lesions, on your intestinal walls. The sigmoidoscopy is only 70% accurate; it is less invasive than the colonoscopy. If there is a history of colorectal cancer in your family, you should opt for the latter.

Colon cancer is treatable if discovered early enough. But we are squeamish about the testing; it involves fasting and purging, as well as some "indignity." (The test itself is done while you are dreamily sedated and doesn't hurt a bit.) But that embarrassment can have a very expensive price tag. Listen to Katie Couric in her drive for colorectal awareness.
Be tested. Be sure.

- Taking medications with simethicone, such as Rolaids®, to ease your distress.
- Swallowing a tablet containing alpha-galactosidase, such as Bean-O®, before eating any gassy foods. It really works!

The Dirt on Diverticulitis

The walls of your large intestines can develop small pouches, or bumps, called diverticula. You usually won't even be aware of them; they are like the wallpaper in your kitchen that you see every day and barely notice. But if they become inflamed or infected—usually from a poor, low-fiber diet or from chronic

constipation—you can develop diverticulitis, which causes severe stomach cramps, nausea, and soreness.

The best treatment, as with so many other gastrointestinal diseases, is a *healthy, high-fiber diet.* This will not only prevent the constipation associated with diverticulitis, it can prevent the pain of the disease itself.

Antibiotics and antispasmodics are usually prescribed to reduce the inflammation and discomfort of diverticulitis.

For more information about gastrointestinal diseases, contact:

Crohn's & Colitis Foundation of America
386 Park Avenue South
New York, NY 10016
(212) 685-3440
(800) 932-2423
(212) 779-4098 (fax)
infoeccfa.org

Digestive Disease National Coalition
711 2nd Street NE, Suite 200
Washington, DC 20002
(202) 544-7497
(202) 546-7105 (fax)
www.ddnc.org

National Digestive Diseases Information Clearinghouse
2 Information Way
Bethesda, MD 20892
(301) 907-8906
www.niddk.nih.gov/health/digest/digest.htm

American Dietetic Association
216 West Jackson Boulevard
Chicago, IL 60606
(312) 899-0040
www.eatright.org

We've now put away the pots and pans, the kitchen aids that make our home and hearth hum. We have finished our tour of our "house," the mind and body that make us vital and strong—at any age.

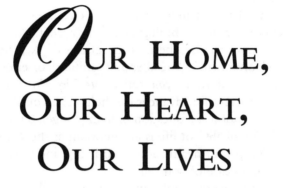

OUR HOME,
OUR HEART,
OUR LIVES

I sing the body electric.
—Walt Whitman

The Baby Boomer's Guide to Women's Health is almost at an end. We have explored the ways our bodies age, the theories and advances that have kept us young in ways our ancestors could only call science fiction.

Surgery that can repair old, worn valves in the heart?

Exercises that can help maintain our mental acuity?

Pills that can keep our sex drive strong?

Strange but true.

But medicine is more than "take a pill and call me in the morning." Today, we know that you must work *with* the miracles of science and technology. Medication alone is not the answer. You must take charge of your life and keep it well.

This means, above all else, a healthy lifestyle. Time and again, throughout this book, a high-fiber, low-fat diet is mentioned as a preventative. Exercise is exalted as a way to keep heart disease, depression, and more at bay. Stress-reduction is a powerful curative for anxiety, memory loss, gastrointestinal disease, and countless other conditions.

We have taken a tour of our house and "viewed" all the rooms of our body: the brain, the circulatory system, the skin and the eyes, the bones and the muscles and the ears. We have discovered the visible signs of aging—and the not so visible symptoms of growing old.

We have learned what we can change—and what, because of genetics or simple biology, we must accept.

Above all else, the message of this book is health. Use it as a "welcome mat," a "needlepoint sampler," or emblazoned on a tee shirt in a drawer: *you can be healthy*. And medicine and the newest scientific advances can help keep you that way.

It is not just a question of living longer, but how well you live.

The quality of life is as important as the years.

Keep your health, your well-being, and your sense of joy alive by taking care of yourself.

Change your mind, and your body will get a spring in its step, a glow in the cheek, a sparkle in the eye.

Change your body, and your mind will feel stronger, more confident. Younger.

A healthy home is a happy home.

To your happy home and a long, fulfilling life.

To your health!

INDEX

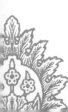

ABOUT THE AUTHORS

Karla Dougherty is a leading writer in the fields of medicine, health, and nutrition. She has authored or co-authored more than 30 books, including *The Spark: The Revolutionary 3-Week Fitness Plan That Changes Everything You Know About Exercise, Weight Control, and Health; The Rockport Walking Program; Living with Brain Injury: A Guide for Families; Living with Stroke: A Guide for Families;* and *Beyond Please and Thank You: A Disability Awareness Handbook for Families, Co-workers, and Friends.* Ms. Dougherty is also the senior writer of HealthSouth Press.

Richard C. Senelick, MD, is the medical director at HealthSouth Rehabilitation Institute of San Antonio (RIOSA). A native of Illinois, Dr. Senelick completed his undergraduate and medical school training at the University of Illinois in Chicago. A neurologist who specializes in neurorehabilitation, he subsequently completed his neurology training at the University of Utah in Salt Lake City. Dr. Senelick has authored numerous publications, including co-authoring *Living with Brain Injury: A Guide for Families, The Spinal Cord Injury Handbook for Patients and Their Families,* and *Living with Stroke: A Guide for Families.* Dr. Senelick is also editor-in-chief of HealthSouth Press.